ASES

A message from the medical editor

Since 2007, our *Annual Report on Prostate Diseases* has provided comprehensive, insightful coverage of the latest developments in prostate research and treatment. Every new issue of the *Annual*, which is geared to the lay audience as well as experts in the field, also contains an interview with a patient.

With this report, we're trying something new: we've compiled a selection of our patient interviews from the past decade, along with updates describing how each of the men we spoke with is doing now. The rationale is simple. After being diagnosed with a prostate disease, men (and their families) often want to know how others with the same condition fared after choosing a particular treatment. This report responds to that need: we learn about the steps men took in selecting a particular therapy, and find out how those treatments affected their long-term health and well-being. Our goal with this report was to assemble a representative sampling of men with varying stages of prostate diseases, with follow-up long enough for our readers to understand the consequences of their treatment decisions.

These interviews cover the most common prostate disorders—prostate enlargement (known medically as benign prostatic hyperplasia, or BPH), which afflicts most men as they get older; prostatitis, which can accompany BPH; and prostate cancer. We also learn how men manage the complications of treatment, such as incontinence and erectile dysfunction. And we speak with wives and partners, to learn more about how a man's prostate disease influences his personal relationships, and how those relationships can in turn help men recover and lead fulfilling lives. With one exception, names and biographical details were changed to protect privacy.

Most of the men we spoke to are pleased with their decisions. Others would have chosen differently knowing what they know now. Our aim with this report is to help men learn from one another, so they can choose a therapeutic approach that fits best with their individual circumstances and lifestyles. More in-depth information about all of these conditions can be found in the *Annual Report on Prostate Diseases*, and this report should be seen as a companion to the *Annual*.

Sincerely,

Marc B. Garnick, M.D.
Medical Editor

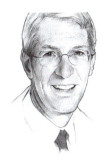

**Medical Editor
Marc B. Garnick, M.D.**

Patient Perspectives *on* PROSTATE DISEASES

Benign prostatic hyperplasia (BPH) with prostatitis: Surgical options

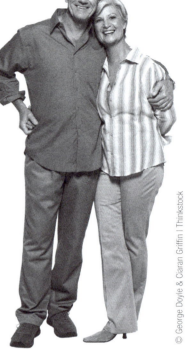

Around the age of 50—and in some cases earlier—a man's prostate starts to grow. This condition, called benign prostatic hyperplasia (BPH), can cause problems with urination because as the prostate gland gets bigger, it compresses and obstructs the urethra, the tube that carries urine from the bladder out of the body. BPH can be treated with medication or surgery. One surgical option, called transurethral resection of the prostate (TURP), involves using specialized tools to remove portions of the obstructing gland to improve urine flow.

In this chapter, we meet two men, Ben Stohr and Robert Bach, who each had a TURP to resolve BPH symptoms. We also meet Ben's wife, Susan.

In addition to BPH, both men had prostatitis, an infection of the prostate that commonly develops in men with BPH. The infection is caused by bacteria that normally live in the colon. The bacteria get on the skin near the anus, multiply there, and then find a way to travel up the urethra to the prostate and bladder. The symptoms come on suddenly and include high fever, chills, joint and muscle aches, and profound fatigue.

Ben and Susan Stohr

In 2013, we interviewed Ben Stohr, a primary care physician, and Susan, his wife of 40 years, about his experience with BPH and TURP to treat the condition. In addition to BPH, Ben also had acute bacterial prostatitis. Following is that 2013 interview.

Q: When did your prostate problems start?
Ben: I am now [in 2013] 66, and my first episode was over 15 years ago, in 1998, when I was 51. I was getting ready to run a 10K road race, and I came down with acute bacterial prostatitis. It was really horrible. I was treated with antibiotics.

Q: What caused the prostatitis?
Ben: Probably benign prostatic hyperplasia—BPH—although that wasn't diagnosed until later. BPH and prostatitis often go hand in hand. With BPH, you don't empty your bladder properly, so if bacteria from the colon get into urine collecting in the bladder, those bacteria can grow and spread to the prostate.

Q: After you were treated for this acute episode, then what happened?
Ben: I had more episodes of prostatitis, and over the years, I was having a little more urinary frequency and urgency, but nothing that was life-shattering. Then in September 2005, about a day after a 30-mile bike race, I peed big blood clots. Even for a physician who has cared for patients with blood in the urine, it was disturbing. I also started peeing tiny little pebbles. So I was diagnosed as having not only BPH, but also bladder stones.

Q: Bladder stones?
Ben: Yes, not kidney stones. Bladder stones are also a consequence of stagnant, concentrated urine. They are little round pellets. You are urinating and then all of sudden, these BBs come out. They aren't necessarily painful like kidney stones are. None of mine got caught coming out. If they had, then that would have been very painful.

I was evaluated completely with a urological evaluation, a cystoscopy to look inside the blad-

Patient Perspectives on PROSTATE DISEASES

der—the whole nine yards. The stones were analyzed, and they were made of uric acid.

Q: *How were the bladder stones treated?*
Ben: With potassium citrate and with allopurinol [Zyloprim], which is a gout medication, because they were uric acid stones. The idea is to decrease the concentration of uric acid in your bladder and in your bloodstream, and to make the pH of the urine more alkaline so uric acid doesn't get a chance to crystallize and form stones.

I was fine for a while, and then I experienced the worst pain of my life.

Q: *Worst pain of your life? What happened?*
Susan: We were all on a family vacation to Florida. He started to feel ill on the airplane, and then when we got there, he got progressively sicker until all of a sudden, it came on full bloom. He was just miserable. Ben had had signs of this illness before, and because he's a physician, he was very aware exactly what was happening on the plane and when we landed.
Ben: Yes, we were celebrating my 60th birthday, and my entire family was there. I went into acute urinary retention, meaning I couldn't pee. It was horrible. We drove to a major medical center nearby where I was catheterized. I had 200 to 300 milliliters [ml] of urine—that's about 10 ounces—and normal retention would be a third of that. Even after they catheterized me, the pain was horrible. My bladder was going into spasm. The spasms would last maybe 20 to 30 seconds and then abate. The pain, on a scale of 1 to 10, was a 12.
Susan: As a physician, Ben knows every complication that could happen, and he understands the development of the disease process. I think it adds to the tension because he knows about all the possible negatives. He knows, "I am going to be given a medicine, and it may or may not work."

Q: *What exactly was the diagnosis and treatment?*
Ben: I had acute prostatitis that led to acute urinary retention in the setting of BPH. I was treated with

antibiotics, the infection abated, and the catheter came out after about a week.

Q: *And the birthday party?*
Susan: Totally ruined. So there was a lot of disappointment.

Q: *So after the acute episode was over, what was the treatment?*
Ben: I started to take BPH medications. I was put on finasteride—Proscar is the brand name—and doxazosin [Cardura], an alpha blocker. And for about a year, I also took daily Cialis [tadalafil], one of the erectile dysfunction [ED] drugs, because Cialis is FDA-approved as treatment for BPH and ED associated with BPH, which I had. [See "Key concepts: Medications for BPH," page 4.]

But as time went on, the urinary frequency was getting worse. So, my entire life revolved around knowing where the bathroom was. It drove Susan crazy.
Susan: Things never returned to normal after that episode in Florida. There was always this concern about future infection and urinary retention. They were never as acute, but Ben did have episodes of infection. He was also taking all those medications—he was a walking pharmacy.

And then the other stress was the constant need to go to the bathroom. So, we always noted where the bathrooms were whenever we went out.

Q: *Sounds frustrating.*
Susan: It was a very difficult period for him and for us. Ben was totally stressed out. Because of the BPH, it took a long time [for Ben to empty his bladder]. It was a process, because he would have to urinate but didn't always have a good stream. We would never leave enough time, and we were always late for everything. And the middle of the night—there was a lot of getting up in the middle of the night.

Q: *And you as a couple were also dealing with ED?*
Susan: Yes, but urination was the biggest day-to-day anxiety.

Patient Perspectives on PROSTATE DISEASES

Key concepts: Medications for BPH

The FDA has approved three types of drugs for BPH:

- Alpha blockers, which help with urination by relaxing certain muscles in the prostate and bladder. Examples include tamsulosin (Flomax) and alfuzosin (Uroxatral).

- 5-alpha-reductase inhibitors, which help reduce the size of the prostate. Examples include dutasteride (Avodart) and finasteride (Proscar). One way to think about the difference between alpha blockers and 5-alpha reductase inhibitors is that alpha blockers help the "going" problem, while 5-alpha-reductase inhibitors help with the "growing" problem.

- The PDE5 inhibitor tadalafil (Cialis), which slows the breakdown of cyclic GMP, a naturally occurring chemical in the body that relaxes smooth muscle (muscle tissue in the penis, gut, and other internal organs that is not under voluntary control). Tadalafil is best known for its effects in the penis, where it improves blood flow during sexual stimulation. It also enhances smooth muscle relaxation in the bladder neck, urethra, and prostate, improving urinary symptoms.

There are also surgical and minimally invasive procedures for treating BPH.

Q: So what made you decide to finally get surgery?

Ben: I had a post-void test, which measures how much urine is in the bladder after you urinate. [See "Key concepts: Post-void residual volume," page 17.] My results showed that after urinating, my bladder wasn't emptying as much as it should. That and the urinary symptoms made me decide to have a procedure done to deal with my BPH. I chose TURP.

Susan: I think it was the surgeon. We had been conferring with him off and on. The surgeon finally said to him, "Ben, it's time." But Ben didn't jump on it. He is not a surgically oriented doctor and will also avoid hospitals at all costs. There were about three more visits before we reached some level of finality.

Q: Ben, why did you pick TURP?

Ben: I considered other surgical alternatives. But redo rates for the alternatives to TURP are really high. I wanted to get as much obstructing prostate tissue out as possible. I wanted to have only one procedure done, probably for the rest of my life, although it's conceivable I may need another one.

Q: What were the first few hours and days after TURP like? How long did it take to recover?

Ben: I went in on day one and got discharged on day two. When you go home, while you're on bed rest, you have to plan on doing absolutely nothing. You just get up to go to the bathroom and to empty the Foley, the bag attached to the catheter. Your urine is bloody and has lots of scary-looking clots in it. Sometimes the urine is clear for a while, and then you pass a clot and it becomes bloody again. Not to worry. It's all part of the healing process.

Bed rest for me lasted for about a week. And I had light ambulation for about another week, and then I went back to work the third week on a half schedule. I would say it took me about three to four weeks to recuperate.

Q: Why is the urine bloody after TURP?

Ben: TURP involves a part of the prostate with a lot of blood vessels. So when the surgeon removes tissue there's a lot of bleeding.

Q: When did you get the catheter out?

Ben: About four to five days after the procedure. They fill up the bladder with 200 to 300 ml of water—again, that's about 10 ounces—then pull out the catheter and see if you can urinate.

Q: And how did that first urination go?

Ben: Great! I had a stream like I was a teenager again.

Q: And how about sexual activity—did that improve?

Susan: Oh, my God. He is like a new man. It's been amazing.

Q: So you're happy with TURP?

Ben: Absolutely! I went off the Proscar, the doxazosin, the potassium citrate, and the Cialis. The only medication I am taking is allopurinol, the gout medication for keeping my uric acid levels down; this should minimize any chance of stones forming again. And I've got to tell you, my life is completely

Patient Perspectives *on* PROSTATE DISEASES

changed. Sometimes it would take me 15 minutes to empty my bladder. I still have to go every few hours, but I can now empty my bladder in 15 to 20 seconds with a real forceful stream.

Also, I don't have the side effects of the medications I was on. The side effects of the medicines are absolutely underreported—especially the sexual side effects: ED and low semen volume. The doxazosin sapped my strength, and the Proscar seemed to sap me of everything else.

Susan: I don't have to worry about leaving the house. I don't have to worry about whether we can plan a big trip. We've got other things to argue about, but we can definitely not argue about being late for things in the same way.

Q: *What advice would you offer to other men and couples?*

Ben: For men who are reading this, I would definitely recommend that you consider having a procedure earlier—well before you find yourself taking medications for BPH for a long time.

Susan: I guess if your issues are more controllable, and you think that the drugs are performing well for you, then I would say continue on that regimen as long as you feel that you're getting an improved result. But for certain men, who are probably at

the extreme—which I think is where Ben ended up—then I think surgery is the right response.

Another thing is that you really have to pick your surgeon very carefully. Even though this seems like a run-of-the-mill operation for a urologist, that may not necessarily be the case. And I think that a lot of Ben's positive results were the result of the surgeon.

Finally, don't rush things during the recovery period. Ben didn't have any of those experiences that could make the recovery a more negative experience.

Q: *And how about running and triathlons?*

Ben: I haven't gone back to biking. My urologist was a little bit hesitant to have me go back to training so hard on a bike. You're sitting right on your prostate gland when you're on a bike, and that causes lots of problems. But I feel great. I am running and swimming. I may even try my first marathon later this year.

2017 update:

Now 70, Ben has since been diagnosed with two cancers that are unrelated to his initial BPH and prostatitis. Treatment for those cancers did affect his sexual functioning. However, he continues to urinate normally after his TURP and believes it was the correct treatment for his BPH.

Robert Bach

Robert Bach gave us an account of his experiences both before and after undergoing TURP for BPH at the age of 71. In his account, he included journal entries for November and December 2011 describing his surgery and his postoperative condition, plus a 2012 entry on his long-term recovery. Following are excerpts.

About five years ago [at the time of writing], I developed recurrent urinary tract infections. My ability to urinate was compromised. I went to a urologist, who diagnosed BPH. I started taking Flomax [tamsulosin] and continued for several years.

Still, the BPH, along with repeated bouts with prostatitis, meant my bladder wouldn't empty all

the way. In January 2009 I consulted a urologist at my local hospital and I decided to switch to Uroxatral [alfuzosin] in place of Flomax and to start taking Proscar [finasteride] to shrink the prostate gland and improve urine flow [see "Key concepts: Medications for BPH," page 4].

The following June, I consulted Dr. Marc Garnick at Beth Israel Deaconess Medical Center because of continuing symptoms of poor bladder drainage. Dr. Garnick performed a full physical exam, including a digital rectal examination [DRE]. He ordered some blood tests, including a prostate-specific antigen [PSA] test [see "Key concepts: PSA," page 10], to look for possible infection or cancer in the prostate.

Patient Perspectives on PROSTATE DISEASES

On June 30, my PSA was 3.14 nanograms per milliliter [ng/ml]. Because the DRE might have caused my PSA to rise, I had another test on July 6, which produced a much better value of 1.78 ng/ml. Still, I consulted Dr. William DeWolf, a surgeon at Beth Israel Deaconess Medical Center, later that month. Because my DRE had some questionable findings, he performed a prostate biopsy of 20 samples on August 5 to rule out cancer. The biopsy found no prostate cancer or precancerous cells.

By this point, the Proscar appeared to be working: my urine flow improved, and my BPH symptoms receded. But in December 2010, some bladder—and possibly prostate—irritation returned and continued into January 2011.

In February, I returned from a trip to Florida with a severe case of flu and developed pneumonia. I started taking one antibiotic, the Z-Pak [azithromycin], and later another antibiotic, Levaquin [levofloxacin], to treat the pneumonia. While I was taking the drugs my bladder irritation improved, which led me to believe that I may have had a low-grade infection of the prostate or bladder.

In March and April the irritation returned, and I consulted my local urologist. He performed urinalysis, urine cytology [a test for abnormal cells coming from the bladder in the urine], ultrasound of my kidneys, and cystoscopy to examine the bladder. Urine cytology showed no evidence of cancerous cells. He prescribed a medication for bladder irritation. I continued to have symptoms of irritation of the bladder or prostate during a 10-day trip in April, and on May 5, I had a blood test to check cholesterol, thyroid, and liver functions. That test also included PSA, which I had not been testing since my negative prostate biopsy in August 2009. The PSA result was 2.99 ng/ml.

On July 14, I consulted Dr. DeWolf about my continuing bladder and prostate irritation and the higher PSA value compared with before. We discussed my having a TURP to promote drainage of the bladder and reduce irritation. At the age of 71, I felt strongly that now was the time to have the procedure.

We scheduled a flow dynamics test, to evaluate how well my urinary system was storing and releasing urine, for October 7. The test demonstrated normal bladder function, but after urinating, I still retained about 200 ml of urine. *[Editor's note: Urine retention amounts in excess of 100 ml are typically associated with BPH, and Robert Bach's were twice that threshold.]* We scheduled a TURP procedure for November 4.

On October 11, I reviewed the procedure to be performed with Dr. DeWolf and had a pre-op meeting with the hospital's anesthesiology department. What follows are some notes I made about what the procedure felt like and how my recovery progressed.

Nov. 4, 2011

I underwent a two-hour bipolar TURP under general anesthesia. *[Editor's note: Bipolar refers to the use of saline fluid to wash away debris during surgery.]* Dr. DeWolf removed the interior tissue of the prostate capsule using a cutting tool and flushed the tissue being removed with a saline solution. He retained the tissue for later pathological examination. The tissue left behind was cauterized with an electrode to minimize bleeding as the area healed. This left a scab, and there was little bleeding after the procedure.

I awoke from the operation with little pain and a catheter in place, which was delivering a flushing saline solution to the bladder, providing antibiotics to prevent infection, and draining the bladder. I was transferred to a hospital room, had no appetite, and spent the rest of the afternoon sleeping. I took no pain medicine, only stool softeners.

Nov. 5, 2011

I was considering having the catheter removed and checking out of the hospital late in the day. Dr. DeWolf was skeptical that one day of recovery would be enough, but agreed to remove the catheter in midafternoon and do a post-void residual test to see if my bladder was performing adequately to avoid urine retention.

Removal of the large post-op catheter was painful so soon after the operation, and urination was painful too. I was unable to expel enough urine, and ultrasound examination showed that I was retaining more urine than I was able to expel. Therefore my doctors determined that I would have a smaller catheter inserted—for drainage only—and would remain in the hospital for another night.

Nov. 6, 2011

I had the option of having the catheter removed and being tested again for urine retention or going home with the catheter in place in order to give my bladder several more days of rest. I chose to return home with the catheter in place. A surgeon at my local hospital would be providing post-op care.

Nov. 7, 2011

While at home, I noticed that the catheter was not draining, and quickly scheduled a visit to my local surgeon's office. He was able to flush out the catheter with saline solution to remove a blood clot blockage from the head of the catheter.

Nov. 9, 2011

After the bladder had two more days of rest, my local surgeon removed the catheter. There was no pain associated with the removal, and after several glasses of water I was able to urinate easily about 1,200 ml over the course of the morning. Dr. DeWolf requested that my local hospital perform an ultrasound post-void residual test that afternoon. The result showed that I was retaining almost no urine in the bladder, and therefore the recovery process was continuing normally.

Nov. 18, 2011

It has been two weeks since the procedure. In the time after the catheter came out, I continued to urinate normally, with little irritation. Blood clots and scab material continued to be flushed out when I urinated. I spent most of the time for the past two weeks either standing or reclined on a couch reading or working on my laptop computer. I slept well at night and took a nap of about an hour each day. I am looking forward to returning to my normal schedule next week, although I do not expect to be feeling 100% for another month.

I learned the pathology report came back with the analysis of the tissue removed during the bipolar TURP—and there is no sign of cancer. That is good to know.

Dec. 16, 2011

During my post-op visit, Dr. DeWolf performed a DRE and examined my urine sample under a microscope. He told me that my white blood cell count was elevated, indicating that healing of the prostate was still under way.

I told Dr. DeWolf that a week earlier I experienced some discomfort while urinating and just afterward. After reviewing my urinalysis results, Dr. DeWolf prescribed an antibiotic.

Dec. 26, 2011

The antibiotic helped, and the discomfort while urinating has disappeared. But I continue to avoid spices and acidic food that in the past have irritated my bladder and urinary tract.

I am very pleased with my ability to urinate easily with a strong stream that allows me to empty my bladder. I would rate my TURP procedure a substantial success.

2012 update

One year later, I am happy to report that the bipolar TURP procedure has made an enormous improvement in the quality of my life. The anxiety of frequent urination is gone. I can enjoy travel and sports without the necessity of planning where I am going to urinate every two hours. My urine stream continues to be strong, and I am emptying my

---

Key concepts: Side effects of TURP

Retrograde ejaculation—in which semen flows into the bladder rather than exiting the body through the penis—affects most men who undergo TURP. The problem develops when the bladder sphincter is destroyed during the procedure. The condition is not harmful, but it may affect fertility (a consideration for younger men).

Impotence, urinary incontinence, infections, and other serious complications occur in about 5% to 10% of men who undergo TURP.

Patient Perspectives *on* PROSTATE DISEASES

2017 update:

Now 79 years old, Robert Bach is still pleased with his decision to undergo TURP for BPH. He has no residual side effects or difficulty urinating and spends much of his time in retirement traveling abroad.

bladder the first time I try to urinate.

During the first three months after the procedure, I continued to feel some sensitivity when urinating. By the fourth month, the area of the prostate that had been cut away had completely healed, and I felt little sensitivity.

Although the TURP procedure made it possible for me to drain my bladder normally and took care of my prostate infections, I still remain susceptible to infection. I experienced a mild prostate infection in early October, upon returning from a strenuous trip to Europe. My doctor prescribed a 10-day course of antibiotics, and the infection went away.

Many men are concerned about what effect a TURP procedure might have on their sexual function. In my case, normal erections returned within

the first three months. The absence of chronic infection certainly contributed to this recovery.

However, I have developed retrograde ejaculation [see "Key concepts: Side effects of TURP," page 7]. When I was taking Uroxatral to relax the sphincter in my bladder, I noticed a reduction in semen ejaculation and a lessening of the sensation during ejaculation. This continued after I underwent TURP. The pleasant sensation of sex up to the point of ejaculation is unaffected by the TURP procedure, but as ejaculation begins I feel a slight burning and warm flow as the ejaculate flows into my bladder. Some of the ejaculate is ejected through my penis. All of this is not to say that the complete sexual experience is compromised, but rather that it is a different experience at the point of ejaculation.

The bottom line is that one year later, I am very happy that I had the TURP procedure and I hope that it will be a permanent fix for me into my 90s. ♥

Patient Perspectives *on* PROSTATE DISEASES

Low-risk prostate cancer: Choosing active surveillance over treatment

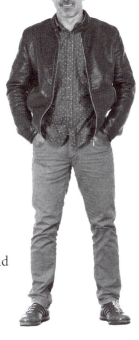

Many prostate cancers grow slowly and do not pose a substantial risk to survival, especially among older men, who are more likely to die of another cause than the cancer. After consulting with their doctors, men who have low-risk prostate cancer may choose to avoid treatment in favor of having their tumors monitored with active surveillance. Men on active surveillance undergo routine digital rectal exams (DREs), tumor biopsies, prostate-specific antigen (PSA) tests, and in some cases, magnetic resonance imaging (MRI) scans of the prostate to check for tumor growth. Treatment is initiated only if and when their tumors begin to spread.

Here, we present the experiences of two men who have each been on active surveillance for more than 20 years. Our first interview is with Jeffrey Caruso, who describes results from his long-term monitoring and the potential triggers that would cause him to seek treatment. We also speak with Benjamin Hunter about the many lifestyle changes he initiated after going on active surveillance.

Jeffrey Caruso

In 1997, when he was 57 years old, Jeffrey Caruso had a PSA test after his physician recommended it as part of his annual check-up. The result—3.9 ng/ml—raised some concern because it fell at the upper end of a normal PSA range of 0 to 4 ng/ml. Jeffrey and his doctor decided to keep testing the PSA to monitor it (see "Key concepts: PSA," page 10).

The next year, Jeffrey's PSA had risen to 4.4 ng/ml. Anxiety set in, and Jeffrey began seeing a urologist, who monitored his PSA and performed DREs. During one of these exams, the urologist noted that a small part of the prostate seemed slightly firmer than the rest, a possible sign of cancer. In 1999, Jeffrey had his first prostate biopsy. It was negative, meaning that it found no cancer.

However, Jeffrey's PSA continued a slow climb. By 2005, it hit 5 ng/ml, and a DRE revealed a pronounced hardening of one area of the prostate. Jeffrey underwent a second biopsy. This one revealed cancer with a Gleason score of 3+3 in a single biopsy core (see "Key concepts: Gleason score," page 11).

At this point, Jeffrey was 65 years old and had tough decisions to make. Our initial interview with him, which follows here, was in 2008. We also include some of his later updates from 2009 and 2014, along with a brief update for 2017.

Q: How did you react to the prostate cancer diagnosis?
Jeffrey: I probably had the same reaction anyone else would: panic and fear. Later, I became depressed, asking "Why me?" I also had a very strong urge to do something immediately. My urologist said that I qualified for surgery and that he could perform the procedure, but that radiation and active surveillance were other options.

Q: But you didn't have surgery to remove the prostate. Why?
Jeffrey: I was ready to at first, but then I went to a radiation oncologist who recommended brachytherapy, which treats cancer by putting radioactive seeds into the prostate. Then another oncologist said that with my early-stage cancer, I could wait

HARVARD MEDICAL SCHOOL   www.health.harvard.edu

Patient Perspectives on PROSTATE DISEASES

Key concepts: PSA

Prostate-specific antigen (PSA) is a protein shed by prostate cells into the bloodstream. PSA levels often rise when a man has prostate cancer, although other conditions also can cause increases in PSA. So PSA is true to its name; it's prostate specific, but it's not cancer specific. That means that a high PSA level can cause a false alarm and lead to unnecessary treatment. For this reason, routine PSA screening in men without symptoms is controversial.

However, PSA testing can be quite useful when monitoring a man who has symptoms, and it is very valuable in gauging whether a particular prostate cancer treatment is working. Surgery and hormonal treatment should both lower PSA levels substantially, and if levels rise after treatment, it could mean these interventions haven't been successful.

up to a year to make a decision. After that I calmed down and started reading a lot about prostate cancer and the available treatments. That's when I became increasingly aware of the potential side effects of various treatments.

Q: Which side effects particularly concerned you?

Jeffrey: I worried most about fecal incontinence, then urinary incontinence, and erectile dysfunction came in third. Even the very best radiation oncologists and surgeons can't guarantee zero side effects.

Q: What other research did you do?

Jeffrey: I read books on prostate cancer, studied raw data and hundreds of scientific papers, looked at websites and online presentations, and attended meetings. What I learned is that there were lots of alternatives, but that no one could say definitively which was best.

Q: So how did you settle on active surveillance?

Jeffrey: It was a very tough decision. But gradually I became convinced that active surveillance presented a reasonable risk. If the cancer had already metastasized, then surgery or radiation wouldn't have helped—the horse would already be out of the barn, so to speak. I hoped that my cancer hadn't metastasized, but I knew it could spread microscopically in ways that weren't detectable with current techniques.

And there were almost no hard data at the time on differences in survival among men undergoing various treatments compared with active surveil-

lance. Prostate cancer typically takes a very long time to grow, and many men diagnosed with it will wind up dying of something else.

Q: Under what circumstances would you stop active surveillance and undergo treatment?

Jeffrey: There are generally accepted criteria for who makes a good active surveillance candidate. The PSA level should be under 10, and mine was 5. Also, PSA levels should rise slowly, and it had taken seven years for mine to rise from 4 to 5, which is incredibly slow. The Gleason score should be less than 7, and mine was 6. I had cancer in fewer than three biopsy cores. As long as you have cancer in only one or two cores, and it's in less than 50% of the core sample, you fit the criteria.

Q: So if your PSA suddenly jumped to 10 ng/ml, would you opt for treatment? Or would you want to see changes in multiple factors before changing course?

Jeffrey: Well, PSA can change for reasons other than prostate cancer. But if my levels doubled within one or two years, that would be a huge red flag that the cancer was advancing. I'd also look at recent biopsy results and Gleason scores. If cancer was found in three or more cores, or in 50% or more of any one core, then I'd consider treatment.

2009 update

Q: How has your condition changed since our interview last year? Are you considering treatment now?

Jeffrey: More than four years have passed since I decided to do active surveillance, and until very recently, my biopsy findings were completely stable. My PSA has barely changed at all.

My fifth—and most recent—biopsy found a little bit more cancer. In the past, I had small amounts of cancer in three cores. This time, there was cancer in four cores. Is that just slightly more of the same tumor or did the tumor actually grow? My doctors don't know for sure, but they suspect there's been some tumor growth, and so according to active sur-

10   HARVARD MEDICAL SCHOOL   www.health.harvard.edu

Patient Perspectives on PROSTATE DISEASES

veillance guidelines, I should logically start to think about treatment.

Q: *What was the percentage of cancer in each of those cores?*
Jeffrey: The percentage in the new core was just below 5%. And there was 10% and 20% respectively in two cores from the right apex and 10% in a core from the right mid-apex. All of the cores were scored a Gleason 3+3.

Institutions use different criteria to determine who's eligible for active surveillance. Some say that you shouldn't have cancer in more than two cores. Some say three or four. At my medical center, it's three cores. But my percentages are relatively low.

Q: *Has your PSA level changed significantly?*
Jeffrey: No, it's held steady. In 2006 it was 5.2, and the most recent reading in 2009 was 5.4. That's given me a certain level of comfort.

Q: *So aside from the question of whether three or four positive cores should be the maximum, you still meet your center's other criteria for pursuing active surveillance.*
Jeffrey: Right. It's best not to have any cancer, but prostate cancer sometimes takes so long to grow that you can outlive it. Mine doesn't seem to be aggressive.

Q: *How is your state of mind? Have you been feeling any stress or panic because of the changes in your condition?*
Jeffrey: No, not at all. When I was first diagnosed, I panicked. But that lasted only a few months. I spent a lot of time studying and getting comfortable with what I knew about my illness and the pros and cons of various treatments. Eventually I started to scale back on that research, and my wife encouraged me in that. She said, "You can't just think about this every day. You've got to get back to real life." Now, I'm used to having prostate cancer, and most of the time, I don't think about it. Also, I know that I'm not alone in this. One in every six men my

age has or will be diagnosed with prostate cancer, and a lot of men don't even know they have it because they don't have symptoms.

2014 update
Q: *Nine years after your cancer diagnosis, you are still on active surveillance, which is a reasonable option for low-risk prostate cancer. How have you monitored your cancer over the years?*
Jeffrey: I've had regular PSA tests. And I've had five biopsies.

Q: *Has your PSA level changed significantly?*
Jeffrey: In 2004, my PSA was slightly over 4. Now it's in the range of 7 to 8, or nearly double after about 10 years. And so to the extent that PSA changes reflect cancer growth, my cancer appears to be stable and slow-growing.

Q: *And PSA tests? How often do you get those?*
Jeffrey: I have a PSA test every three months or so. If it doubles in two or three years, then the doctors get worried, and I would get worried too.

Q: *What have your biopsies shown?*
Jeffrey: I haven't had a biopsy since 2009.

Q: *Why not?*
Jeffrey: Well, I had 100 cores from all my prior biopsies combined and only a few contained cancer. So I feel like we know more or less where things stand. And the more biopsies you have, the greater your risk of erectile dysfunction, urinary problems, and infection. So I told my doctors I don't want

---

Key concepts: Gleason score

The Gleason score, which indicates the aggressiveness of a prostate tumor, assigns a number ranging from 2 to 10 to the tumor. It is calculated by grading cell growth patterns for the two most common types of cancer cells in a biopsy specimen and then adding them together. The slowest growing cells are assigned a score of 1 and the fastest growing cells are assigned a score of 5. Thus, if the two most common cell types in a biopsy specimen each have a grade of 3, then the Gleason score is 3+3=6. Prostate cancers with a Gleason score of 6 or below are considered low risk, especially for men with an expected life span of 10 years or less, while cancers with a Gleason score of 7 or higher are considered more aggressive and require treatment.

Patient Perspectives on PROSTATE DISEASES

another one unless there was a compelling reason, like my PSA jumps from 8 to 20.

Q: *What did they suggest instead of a biopsy?*
Jeffrey: A biopsy remains the gold standard for detecting cancer, no question. But when I said "stop," my doctors suggested we follow up with an MRI scan, which provides clear images of the prostate non-invasively. Monitoring prostate cancer progression with MRI is not a generally accepted medical technique right now. Some physicians are doing it with some patients by mutual agreement.

The MRI is noninvasive. But it's not a very pleasant thing. You go into a tube, and there's loud noise, like the pinging submarine noise in movies. And even though they give you something to cover your ears, you still hear it. And you have to lie there for close to an hour. And they tell you don't move, of course, which is very hard. Plus, it's endorectal MRI, which uses something like a mini antenna inserted into the rectum, inside a balloon. The balloon is blown up when it's inside. It's pretty uncomfortable, but at least you're not running a risk of infection, because your skin is not broken. I had my first MRI scan in 2005, another in 2008, and a third in 2012. None revealed any progression beyond what the earlier biopsies had shown, so that was reassuring.

Q: *And digital rectal exams?*

2017 update:

Now 78 years old, Jeffrey has never been treated for his prostate cancer. His latest PSA reading, in 2017, was 9.4 ng/ml.

Jeffrey: Twice a year. The doctor will try to feel if the tumor is getting bigger and approaching the outer edge of the prostate capsule, which is a worrisome development. It helps to have the same doctor do it every time so he or she has some background on your gland.

Q: *You've been on active surveillance now for nine years. How are you feeling about it?*
Jeffrey: Not disturbed. I use a football analogy to describe it. Surgery and radiation are like long field passes—you might get a touchdown, but maybe not. Active surveillance is more like moving the ball with short passes. You keep an eye on the cancer with PSA tests, DREs, and MRI scans. I'm not going to throw a long pass unless something changes and I have to.

Q: *Have you changed anything about the way you eat or behave?*
Jeffrey: I took selenium when I was first diagnosed. And then various other studies have come out saying these supplements don't do anything. *[Editor's note: The SELECT study in 2014 showed that selenium supplements can actually* increase *the risk of high-grade prostate cancer.]* I just dropped all the supplements. I have been active all my life. I still play tennis and swim. I exercise three or four hours a day. And in Florida, I go out and bike with my wife. Twenty miles is our standard trip.

Q: *What advice do you have for a man newly diagnosed with prostate cancer?*
Jeffrey: Don't panic, and don't do the first thing that comes to mind. It's normal to panic when you hear the word "cancer," but prostate cancer is different. Find out what your test results are. If the pathology report shows your cancer is Gleason 6, and you've got a PSA under 10, and the doctor can't feel a tumor during a DRE, then you've probably got a slow-growing cancer and plenty of time to decide what to do.

Patient Perspectives on PROSTATE DISEASES

Benjamin Hunter

In 1996, when Benjamin Hunter was in his mid-50s, he was much like any other man at that stage of life: He was married with children, felt generally healthy, and had no real urinary difficulties. He tried to exercise when he could and ate a typical American diet. Having spent two years in California working on a film, Benjamin returned to his home on the East Coast and contacted his doctor to schedule a routine physical exam. His routine was about to be disrupted.

While doing a digital rectal exam, Benjamin's internist felt something on his prostate gland that she described as an "anomaly"—not entirely normal, but not suggestive of cancer, either. She recommended a PSA test, which revealed that his PSA was 5.7 ng/ml. He subsequently underwent a prostate biopsy. One of the cores removed during the biopsy contained cancer, with a Gleason score of 3+3. He underwent a bone scan and a CT scan to check for signs of metastasis, but there was no evidence the cancer had spread.

Benjamin sought advice from several doctors. Almost every physician he consulted suggested that he undergo traditional treatment with either a radical prostatectomy (surgery to remove the prostate, seminal vesicles, and nearby lymph nodes) or some form of radiation therapy. After giving the matter much thought and doing extensive research, he instead decided on a strategy of active surveillance. In this 2006 interview, he explains why.

At the time of our interview, it was 10 years after his initial diagnosis. He was 64 years old and was working as a film writer and director. He was also actively involved in various philanthropies.

Q: _Can you share some of the emotions and thoughts you had while dealing with your diagnosis?_
Benjamin: At first, I was fearful. I couldn't sleep at night. I was worried about the future.

Q: _What type of research did you do, as you evalu-_

ated treatment options? And what information most affected your decision?
Benjamin: I started to gather information and seek out other opinions about what I should do. What amazed me was that there were many choices, but no clear indication of which was best. I could choose from radical prostatectomy, traditional radiation, radioactive seeds, freezing the prostate, burning the prostate—there were all these different options. The doctors presented the pros and cons of each one and recommended that I think about it carefully and then decide what I wanted to do.

Nobody rushed me. The doctors all said this was a slow-growing cancer and that I could take a month or two to investigate and decide which way to go. But nobody suggested the option of active surveillance. At the time, that type of strategy was normally reserved for people who were a lot older than I was, or people who had some other serious medical condition that would make treatment too risky.

As it happens, my wife does occasional research about medical conditions for friends. So she helped me do research on the Internet as well as in books, to learn more about the disease so that I could try to make a treatment decision.

And what bothered me was that, literally in the first month that I was thinking about this, I started to hear anecdotes about other men in my position. I heard about one acquaintance who had surgery for prostate cancer, suffered adverse consequences, and then his cancer had come back. So that made me wonder how effective the treatments were. Those anecdotal pieces of evidence were very profound, because you'd think, "Wow, what if that happened to me? That would be a terrible outcome." So I decided to really research and think things through carefully before doing anything.

Q: _It sounds as if the side effects of treatment were most bothersome to you, and might have had the most impact on your decision. Is that accurate?_
Benjamin: I know some men with prostate cancer think, "Do whatever it takes to cure me of this dis-

Patient Perspectives on PROSTATE DISEASES

ease." For me, it was more a matter of weighing the risks and benefits.

At the time, what most hit me were the side effects of treatment. The doctors told me that with surgery there was a 30% chance of impotence, and maybe a 5% chance of incontinence. That's a pretty stunning thing to hear, when you consider yourself in the prime of life and healthy. But radiation wasn't any better. It had similar complications, with slightly different percentages, but it might also cause rectal damage. So I continued to research the various options and compare the numbers.

It became clear that the various treatments had slightly different side effect profiles, but not meaningfully different. So then it became a question of, if I'm going to face these side effects, what are the chances that a treatment will actually improve my health or my longevity? And what I found out was that there was no information that proved that any of these treatments would actually lengthen my life. So that really struck me. It was all risk and no guarantee of benefit.

Q: *You've made some significant lifestyle changes. Can you talk about why you thought this was so important?*

Benjamin: From my research, I knew that in Japan, prostate cancer was very rare. I came across an autopsy study comparing men who died in auto accidents in either Japan or the United States. It found that the number of precancerous prostate lesions was about the same in both groups. And yet the prevalence of prostate tumors is much higher in America than it is in Japan. But when Japanese men move to America, after a generation or two, their prostate cancer rates are the same as American men's. So this led me to hypothesize that prostate cancer is a lifestyle disease.

This raised the possibility that if I could change my lifestyle, then perhaps I could combat the disease. So I saw lifestyle change as a two-prong strategy: it might inhibit new tumors from emerging, while slowing the growth of existing tumors.

The slow-growing nature of these tumors also meant that there was always the chance that I would die from another disease or accident without facing the terrible side effects from prostate cancer treatment. And new treatments might emerge, such as a cancer vaccine. So in some ways I decided to play for time. In the end, I made about 50 lifestyle changes in response to having cancer.

Q: *What dietary changes did you make?*

Benjamin: I am now a vegetarian. I try to eat food that is as close as possible to the source, such as whole grains. And I pay attention to the science. For instance, one study came out of Harvard about the benefit of eating cooked tomatoes, which reduces the risk of prostate cancer. So now I eat seven to 10 servings of cooked tomatoes per week in foods like spaghetti sauce and so on. For the past decade I have not eaten any kind of animal meat whatsoever. But I usually eat fish twice a week, for the omega-3 fats, which laboratory studies have shown may slow tumor growth. Each day, I drink one glass of red wine and have at least three cups of green tea—for the antioxidants, which limit cell damage.

I don't eat dairy products or eggs. I've had almost no refined sugar in the past decade. I'll have about one oatmeal raisin cookie a month, as an occasional indulgence.

One good thing about this diet: I've lost at least 10 pounds. And that's important because I learned early on that keeping my weight down might protect against the development and progression of cancer.

Q: *What other sorts of changes have you made in your lifestyle?*

Benjamin: I work on stress reduction. I now do yoga and go for massage therapy. I exercise about four times a week. And I try to take time to "smell the flowers," as they say, and take walks in the woods.

I also take a COX-2 inhibitor, Celebrex [celecoxib], every day, because it may be helpful in keeping the cancer at bay. [*Editor's note: That was current*

Patient Perspectives *on* PROSTATE DISEASES

treatment at the time of this interview, but would not be recommended today.]

So I've really collected information from multiple sources, and then I evaluate the source. So, for example, if I read about a Harvard study, I figure that's pretty reliable. But if someone is promoting something and I've never heard of it or them, I might look for information elsewhere and ask some people I respect before trying it.

Q: *How often do you monitor your PSA levels? And what other evaluations do you undergo to make sure the cancer is not advancing?*

Benjamin: I get my PSA tested every three or four months—it's risen from about 5.7 to 12.2 since I was diagnosed. I see my oncologist about once every nine or 10 months and occasionally have some tests to see if there's any indication of spread. I've decided to avoid prostate biopsies. First of all, they hurt. Second, I believe the biopsies have risks. And third, there's no information that I would receive from a biopsy that would cause me to do anything differently.

Q: *Your PSA levels have been elevated a few times, and you've found that these increases correlate with travel. Can you describe your experience with this?*

Benjamin: A few times, my PSA has spiked. One time, it went from 8.6 to 11.7. Another time, it went from 8.9 to 12.0. I suspect it has to do with lifestyle changes during travel. On probably four occasions, when I traveled to India and then had a PSA test after my return, we found the PSA jumped. I think that's because of a combination of stresses. First of all, just sitting in an airplane for 10 or 12 hours is hard on the body, not to mention traveling through all those time zones. And when I travel like that, I tend to get off my regimen. I'll eat vegetarian food, but it may not be exactly what I would eat at home. I don't get massages or practice other stress-reduc-

tion techniques. But so far, once I've been home for a while, my PSA levels stabilize or come back down to where they were.

Q: *What would have to change for you to consider being treated more traditionally? And what would you do?*

Benjamin: If my PSA started to shoot up significantly, or stayed elevated, then I would talk to my doctor about how I might use hormonal treatments to keep the disease at bay. *[Editor's note: Hormonal treatments suppress testosterone, a hormone that makes prostate cancer grow faster.]* I consider hormonal treatment something to keep in my "gunnysack," because although it involves side effects, for the most part they're not permanent. Of course, before making a decision, I'd evaluate the known risks.

Q: *Few people in 1996 decided on active surveillance. Knowing what you do now, would your treatment selection be the same?*

Benjamin: I know active surveillance isn't for everyone. I just know that for me, this was the right choice. I'd make the same choice today that I did 10 years ago. But I'd be less afraid, and I'd be more decisive.

Q: *Any other thoughts?*

Benjamin: This is sincere: Cancer caused me to clean up my life. Today I feel better, I'm living healthier, and because of the lifestyle changes I've made, I've reduced my risk of heart attack, stroke, and other diseases. At least according to the actuarial tables, I'm going to live longer. So I've actually benefited from having this disease. ♥

2017 update:

Now 75 years old, Benjamin Hunter is in his 22nd year on active surveillance. His prostate gland has increased in size and his PSA level ranges up to 50 ng/ml—a high level, but one that has risen very slowly over the years. He has never had another prostate biopsy. He has chronic but stable urinary symptoms and no evidence of metastatic prostate cancer.

Patient Perspectives *on* PROSTATE DISEASES

Low-risk prostate cancer: Choosing treatment

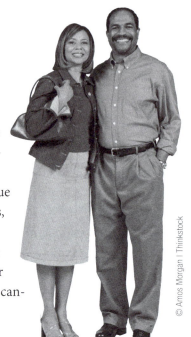

Active surveillance can be an option for some men with low-risk prostate cancer, but it's not appropriate for everyone, and some men feel uncomfortable allowing cancer to remain in the body. In this chapter, we hear from two men who opted for treatment. Every man's decision depends on his unique circumstances, and that's certainly true of our first interviewee, Kirby Parsons, whose decision to have a radical prostatectomy—which involves removing the entire gland—was motivated as much by a need to resolve his debilitating BPH symptoms as by the cancer. We also hear from Brian Kols, who opted for a newer surgical procedure called targeted focal therapy, which removes only cancerous portions of the prostate while leaving the rest of the gland intact.

Kirby Parsons

Kirby Parsons had suffered for years with BPH symptoms that often woke him repeatedly at night; he had trouble urinating and felt as though his bladder never completely emptied. After his PSA level shot up from 2.8 ng/ml to 13.9 ng/ml in just six months, Kirby, who is a doctor, suspected a recent bout of prostatitis was the cause. When medication to treat the prostatitis and ease the symptoms of BPH didn't lower his PSA by as much as expected, he reluctantly had a prostate biopsy. The results showed small amounts of low-grade prostate cancer.

Kirby could have pursued active surveillance. Instead, he opted for a radical prostatectomy, which took place in December 2009, when he was 58 years old. Why didn't he try active surveillance? Did the prostatectomy relieve his urinary symptoms? Does he have any regrets about his treatment decision? In this 2010 interview, Kirby shared his thoughts on these questions.

Q: What symptoms of BPH did you have, and how long had you been experiencing them?
Kirby: I probably started having urinary symptoms six or seven years ago. I was getting up several times a night to urinate, but felt like I couldn't fully empty my bladder, and the symptoms were worse when I was traveling. I had also had a couple of episodes of prostatitis; one of them actually occurred after a long trip. It was remarkably uncomfortable—dribbling, groin and abdominal pain, and fever.

Q: What was your PSA at that point?
Kirby: We didn't do a PSA then because it would have been overly high due to the infection. But shortly after the prostatitis, I did have my PSA measured and it was 13.9. My PSA about six months before that was 2.8. I was almost 57 years old at the time.

Q: Is there any history of prostate trouble in your family?
Kirby: My father had both BPH and prostate cancer. He was treated with hormonal therapy and radiation and died of Alzheimer's disease at age 80.

Q: When did you start taking medication for BPH?
Kirby: I started taking Flomax [tamsulosin] in 2004 or 2005. It didn't really work, so we increased the dose. After the episode of prostatitis, my urologist recommended taking Avodart [dutasteride], too, so I started taking that in December 2007. [See "Key concepts: Medications for BPH," page 4.] It affected my libido, and my semen volume seemed to go

Patient Perspectives *on* PROSTATE DISEASES

down. And I didn't like how it made me feel. Also, I was always worried that I might run out of medication when traveling and go into acute urinary retention.

Q: Did that ever happen?
Kirby: No, but I'm sure I came close.

Q: What was your understanding of what should happen to your PSA when you started taking Avodart?
Kirby: I knew it should fall by about 50%, but I was a little unclear about where the 50% mark was, given that my PSA rose so high with the episode of prostatitis. Should it be 50% down from 13.9 or from 2.8?

I actually put off having my PSA remeasured because I was concerned about what the results would be. With a family history of prostate cancer, I expected to be diagnosed with it someday.

Q: So how did your urologist convince you to have a biopsy?
Kirby: Well, my BPH symptoms were really getting uncomfortable. My post-void residual volume was about 125 ml, just above the amount that defines chronic urinary retention. [See "Key concepts: Post-void residual volume," above right.] I was already on the maximum dose of Flomax, and I had been on Avodart for about a year. When the PSA was measured at that point at 2.7, we felt it really hadn't fallen adequately. Given my PSA level, family history, and symptoms, I knew I needed a biopsy.

Q: What was that experience like?
Kirby: With some local anesthesia and a mild sedative beforehand, it was not nearly as bad as I had feared. It was quick, and it was not particularly painful.

Q: What were the findings of the biopsy?
Kirby: The pathology was abnormal in two of the 20 cores, so 18 cores showed no evidence of cancer.

The cancer we did find was in 5% of the two cores, and it had a Gleason score of 3+3.

Interestingly, ultrasound showed my prostate volume was 61 cubic centimeters [cc], which is relatively large, even after taking Adovart for a year. Avodart is supposed to shrink the prostate, but after a year, my prostate went from 60 to 61 cc, even though I didn't miss a dose.

> ### Key concepts: Post-void residual volume
>
> Post-void residual volume refers to the amount of urine remaining in the bladder after a man tries to empty it. Amounts in excess of 100 ml are generally associated with BPH.

Q: Given the nature of your cancer, you could have opted for active surveillance. Why did you decide to have a radical prostatectomy?
Kirby: The way I viewed it, and the way my urologist viewed it, was that I was uncomfortably symptomatic with BPH and lower urinary tract symptoms. I was on the maximum doses of medications that were supposed to control the symptoms, but they weren't working. So I needed a procedure to reduce the size of my prostate, such as a TURP, TUEVP [transurethral electrovaporization of the prostate, which uses a heated electrode to vaporize tissue], or laser surgery. But would having one of those procedures make sense for someone with prostate cancer? I didn't think so.

Radiation therapy would probably make my prostate more inflamed, increasing the odds that I would experience acute urinary retention. And I would have had to take hormones to shrink my prostate prior to radiation, which I didn't want to do. I was also an inappropriate candidate for brachytherapy [radioactive seeds implanted in the prostate through the rectum to deliver radiation internally] because my prostate was larger than the general threshold of 50 cc.

That left me with two choices: have no treatment and continue to put up with the urinary symptoms, or treat the cancer, and thus the BPH and the urinary symptoms, with a radical prostatectomy. I decided that the radical prostatectomy would be the best thing for me.

HARVARD MEDICAL SCHOOL   www.health.harvard.edu

Patient Perspectives on PROSTATE DISEASES

Q: Did you look into the various types of radical prostatectomy—laparoscopic, robotic, and open?
Kirby: I did, and I decided to have the open surgery. Based on what I read at that time, robotic surgery didn't really seem to have a proven benefit.

Q: If you hadn't had urinary problems, what treatment would you have had?
Kirby: Without urinary symptoms, I would have been leaning toward active surveillance.

Q: Even with your family history?
Kirby: That was the one piece that made me uncomfortable with active surveillance.

Q: What was the postoperative period and recovery like?
Kirby: I had a hard time the first two days after surgery because the painkillers caused nausea and stomach upset. After a medication change, I was much more comfortable. I was in the hospital for three-and-a-half days, and after I went home, I didn't really need any pain medication. The one medication that I did use was for sleep—I found that I was able to sleep comfortably despite having the catheter in place.

I didn't really leave the house until I went to the hospital to have the catheter removed, which was about nine or 10 days after surgery. I went back to work part-time after about three weeks.

Q: Presumably, you've stopped taking Flomax and Avodart. How is your urinary function now?
Kirby: I stopped taking Flomax and Avodart the day of the surgery. And from the day the catheter was removed, I haven't had any significant urinary symptoms—no diminished flow or feelings of obstruction. In fact, the change in how quickly and completely I can empty my bladder has been dramatic.

Q: How have you felt since undergoing surgery, and are you pleased with the outcome?
Kirby: My first goal was to be cancer-free, but not far behind that was my desire to take care of the

BPH and have the urinary symptoms under control. The downsides to surgery for me—urinary incontinence, leakage, and sexual function—were much less important. Clearly, the cancer has been taken care of. My PSA is undetectable, and I'm not at risk for a recurrence. I have no problems with urinary flow or incontinence. I was on another trip not that long ago and, as opposed to the trips where I was the first one in the bathroom and the last one out, I'm now the first one out.

Leakage has not been a significant issue. Initially, there was a little bit, so I wore pads. Now, if I'm going to be out of reach of a bathroom for long periods of time, I'll wear a pad just in case, but more than 90% of the time, I haven't needed it. And I don't wear a pad at night.

Erectile dysfunction is still an issue, but I had surgery only eight months ago, so the jury is still out on that. Doctors say it can take 18 months to two years to recover erectile function. As of now, that's the only issue I'm still dealing with.

I will say that since I stopped taking Flomax, I haven't had the lightheadedness and dizziness that I used to get. And having stopped Avodart, my libido is a little better.

Q: What advice do you give your male patients who are in a similar situation?
Kirby: I have quite openly shared my own experience with my patients. Before my treatment, I kept things very private, but afterward, I've almost felt obligated to discuss my experience. I tell people with prostate cancer that, unlike with other types of cancer, there's no single approach to treatment. Every man's story is unique. You can't say, "Well, this man had brachytherapy, so that's what I'm going to do," or "My friend is doing active surveillance, so that's what I'm going to do." Treatment really has to be individualized, much more so than with other malignancies. I've told people that they need to recognize the uniqueness of their own situation.

I also recommend that people gather as much information as they can about various therapies and be thoughtful about their treatment choice. I know

Patient Perspectives on PROSTATE DISEASES

that people can become paralyzed by information because when you do research on the Internet or talk to people, there's always one more thing to consider. But my advice is to get as much information as you can, focus on the things that are most important to you and prioritize them, and then think about how the various therapies fit with your priorities.

Q: *As a physician, you probably knew a lot about prostate cancer before you even started to study your own situation. Could you have become paralyzed by all of that information?*
Kirby: Yes, I think so. As a physician, there's an expectation of understanding things to an even

greater level. You look through all the levels of nuance and think through experimental data. It could really derail one's ability to focus on making a decision. Many people gave me information or suggested talking to yet another doctor at a hospital across the country. After a while, all of that information could have been paralyzing. That's why you have to focus on your priorities, what makes you comfortable, and the uniqueness of your own situation.

2017 update:

Now 66 years old, Kirby Parsons is pleased with his decision to have a radical prostatectomy. However, his erectile function, while improved, never returned to its pre-surgery level.

Brian Kols

In March 2010, Brian Kols, 59, had recently been diagnosed with prostate cancer. Doctors recommended radical prostatectomy, but Brian was concerned about the side effects. He sought a second opinion from Dr. David Crawford, professor of surgery, urology, and radiation oncology and head of the Section of Urologic Oncology at the University of Colorado Anschutz Medical Campus, in Denver. Dr. Crawford recommended a different course of action. Instead of treating the whole prostate gland with surgery or radiation, he pointed Brian toward a newer option called targeted focal therapy, which offers a compromise solution. With targeted focal therapy, doctors treat only cancerous portions of the prostate while leaving the rest of the gland—including the nerves that control erectile and bowel function and the muscles that control urinary continence—intact. Targeted focal therapy can be performed in a number of ways. Doctors can freeze tumor tissue with cryotherapy, or they can destroy it with high-intensity focused ultrasound (which uses sound waves to selectively heat tumors to lethal temperatures while sparing normal tissue).

Harvard-affiliated hospitals do not offer targeted focal therapy for prostate cancer. Therefore, in this 2015 interview, we spoke with both Brian Kols and Dr. Crawford.

Q: *Dr. Crawford, would you please introduce Brian and describe his case?*
Dr. Crawford: I first met Brian in March of 2010, when he sought us out for an opinion on his prostate cancer, which had been diagnosed a few months earlier. At the time, he was 59 years old. A biopsy had revealed Gleason 6 cancer in 10% of a single core on one side of his prostate. He didn't have a markedly elevated PSA level, and his prostate volume was 45 cubic centimeters [cc]. Other doctors had recommended radical prostatectomy, but Brian was newly married and concerned about the sexual side effects. And apart from his cancer, he was the picture of health and a nonsmoker. The rectal exam didn't raise any significant concerns, although there had been some urinary bleeding that was attributed to a separate bladder tumor, which was successfully treated in a separate procedure.

So his case brings home the whole issue of overdiagnosis and overtreatment of prostate cancer. For 20 years patients have been asking me, "Hey Doc, why can't you just take out part of my prostate, or why can't I have a lumpectomy like some women with breast cancer?" We would explain that prostate cancer exists in multiple places in the gland, and that 20% to 30% of men diagnosed with low-grade disease actually harbor

HARVARD MEDICAL SCHOOL www.health.harvard.edu

Patient Perspectives *on* PROSTATE DISEASES

something worse that's been missed on biopsy. That's what got us to start doing mapping biopsies, which take dozens of cores from the prostate in a tight grid. We use the results to generate a three-dimensional model of the gland, and we don't miss any significant cancer that way—our assessment of the prostate is as good as if we had taken the gland out. When we did a mapping biopsy on Brian, we found he was in a very good position for a partial ablation [targeted tissue destruction] that would save his nerves and preserve his sexual potency.

Q: Brian, let's turn it over to you now. What led up to your diagnosis of prostate cancer?

Brian: It started with my PSA history. The first time I had it checked was in August of 2005, and the level was 2.1. Then in 2007 it went up to 4.2, and in April 2009 it was 6.49. I also had microscopic amounts of blood in my urine, so my general practitioner recommended that I see a urologist. I had a biopsy at the urologist's office, and that's when we found the cancer.

I was given three options: one would be to monitor the cancer with active surveillance, another was to have a radical prostatectomy, and the third option was radiation. Active surveillance didn't interest me because my PSA was changing so fast—I knew that I would always be wondering when the cancer was going to flare up. And the consequences of radical treatment worried me, especially radical prostatectomy and the possibility of erectile dysfunction. I kept thinking, "There has got to be a better option, something in between." And that's what brought me to Dr. Crawford.

Q: Do you have a family history of prostate cancer, Brian?

Brian: Not that I'm aware of, no.

Q: Was your family involved in your decision to go with focal therapy?

Brian: Absolutely. My wife found Dr. Crawford on the Internet.

Q: What were your initial thoughts about focal therapy as opposed to the other options you were hearing about?

Brian: I was encouraged that it could have fewer side effects than traditional surgery, and that we could always take the prostate out later if the cancer kept growing. The way I saw it, focal therapy kept my options open.

Dr. Crawford: Brian had been eligible for active surveillance based on one biopsy containing Gleason 6 cancer. Then we performed a mapping biopsy that showed more extensive disease, including a bit of pattern 4 [which raised his overall Gleason score to 3+4, or Gleason 7].

Q: Dr. Crawford, how many places in the country have the same type of focal therapy program that you have? I know some centers no longer do mapping biopsies because of complications with infections.

Dr. Crawford: No one does mapping biopsies to the extent that we do them. We mark the location of every snippet of tissue that we take so we know exactly where in the prostate it comes from. Then we use that information to generate a three-dimensional view of where the cancer is so we can target these areas for treatment.

Q: Are the mapping biopsies all transperineal [taken through the skin between the scrotum and the anus], or do you do them transrectally [through the rectum] as well?

Dr. Crawford: We always do them transperineally, and so far we haven't seen any infectious complications. However, we do see infectious complications from the transrectal biopsies that are done in follow-up.

Q: What sort of antibiotic regimen do you use?

Dr. Crawford: We are seeing more serious antibiotic-resistant infections following transrectal prostate biopsies. So in the past 12 months we have intensified our antibiotic coverage to include drugs like levofloxacin [Levaquin], and we are also adding

Patient Perspectives on PROSTATE DISEASES

injections of gentamicin [Garamycin] at the time of the biopsy.

Q: *How do you select which tissues you're going to treat?*

Dr. Crawford: We treat all the cancer that we can see.

Q: *Is the procedure done under general, regional, or local anesthesia?*

Dr. Crawford: We can do it either way, but we mostly do it under general anesthesia since we don't want our patients to move at all.

Q: *What do you tell people to expect after the procedure?*

Dr. Crawford: We tell them that in rare cases they might have some mild, reversible erectile dysfunction that generally lasts for a couple of months. Infections haven't been a problem. Some men have a bit of trouble urinating.

Q: *How long after the mapping biopsy did you have your procedure, Brian?*

Brian: The biopsy was on March 25, 2010, and then I had my targeted therapy a few months later, on July 8.

Dr. Crawford: How did your procedure go, and what were your thoughts when it was over?

Brian: It went well, and I was relieved that my nerves were never cut. However, I did have some discomfort from the catheter, which was in for three or four days.

Dr. Crawford: Which was easier, the mapping biopsy or the focal therapy? Or were they about the same?

Brian: About the same—I'd say the focal therapy was a little easier. I was able to go right back to work.

Dr. Crawford: And how long was the catheter kept in after the focal therapy, as opposed to the biopsy?

Brian: Four days after the biopsy, and three days after the focal therapy. But it was easier the second time around, since I knew what to expect.

Q: *Did you have any side effects?*

Brian: No, not really. My potency was reduced a little bit for the first three months. But Dr. Crawford said it would return, and sure enough, it did—I'm now as good as ever. I don't need drugs to help with my erections, and I don't have any urinary or bowel problems.

Dr. Crawford: Tell us about the changes in your PSA since we performed the procedure back in 2010.

Brian: My PSA level fell substantially. When I last had it recorded, on Dec. 13, 2014, it was 0.43.

Q: *How much of the prostate was actually treated?*

Dr. Crawford: I would say we took about half. So it's certainly smaller, but not so small that the reduction in size by itself would explain why Brian's PSA level has fallen so low.

Q: *What about additional follow-up?*

Dr. Crawford: Our current approach—and this is subject to change—is to biopsy every year for at least the first couple of years. If results are still negative, then we go to every other year. Brian's tests are still negative at five years, and now we're asking if we really need to do another biopsy if his PSA stays low. But this is uncharted territory.

Q: *What do the treated tissues look like under the microscope?*

Dr. Crawford: A lot of it looks like normal prostate tissue, although we do see some scarring and inflammation. It would be worrisome to see atypical small acinar proliferation [lesions that suggest malignancy], but that hasn't happened with Brian—his biopsies have been fine. But I tell my patients, "You know, you might need another treatment later." About 6% of the men I've treated with focal therapy eventually got a radical prostatectomy. We're pretty particular about who gets focal therapy.

Q: *So, Brian, has the treatment met your expectations?*

HARVARD MEDICAL SCHOOL   www.health.harvard.edu

Patient Perspectives *on* PROSTATE DISEASES

Brian: Oh, I'm very pleased—everything is normal. I should point out that I am on Proscar [finasteride], which is used for BPH, but there's also some evidence that it can help to prevent low-grade cancer [see "Key concepts: Medications for BPH," page 4].

Dr. Crawford: BPH can elevate PSA, so we use Proscar to control for that. If PSA levels rise while a patient is on the drug, it's usually because something significant is happening with his cancer.

2017 update:

Now 67 years old, Brian remains very pleased with his treatment decision. His PSA is low and stable, and he has no incontinence or problems with sexual functioning. He has biopsies every two years.

Q: Who is and who is not a candidate for focal therapy?

Dr. Crawford: Generally someone with small volumes of cancer, usually Gleason 6 or maybe Gleason 3+4 in no more than 20% of cores. It's not for somebody who has 4+3 cancer all around his prostate or bilaterally in a pattern 4—we're talking about low-grade risk. Our intent with the mapping biopsy is to isolate these Gleason 6 and 3+4 cancers and to make sure that there's nothing else there. But we will treat a Gleason 8 cancer if it's located in a small area. So this is really precision medicine. I would say 40 out of 100 patients who walk through our doors with prostate cancer might be eligible for mapping biopsies.

Q: Brian, do you have any parting comments?

Brian: Well, I'm extremely grateful. I have a great quality of life, and I want other men facing a similar situation to know about my experience. ♥

Patient Perspectives *on* PROSTATE DISEASES

High-risk prostate cancer: Undergoing treatment

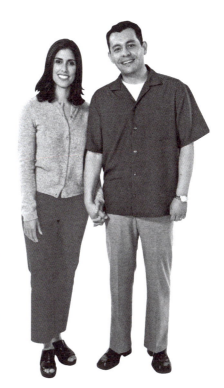

Unlike low-risk prostate tumors, which grow slowly, high-risk prostate cancer poses a more immediate threat to survival. We interviewed two men, Adam Goldstein and Jim Rogers, about their experiences with high-risk prostate cancer. Adam learned he had the disease at a young age, when he was just 45 years old and otherwise in fine health. Jim, a physician, was interviewed together with his wife, Terri, and spoke about how a new technology at the time, endorectal magnetic resonance imaging (MRI), played a decisive role in his treatment decision. Both men were treated with hormonal therapy and radiation.

© Ryan McVay | Thinkstock

Adam Goldstein

In this 2014 interview, Adam, who was 52 at the time we spoke with him, describes his experience with an aggressive Gleason 4+5 (Gleason 9) prostate cancer, and treatment with hormone-blocking drugs and radiation. Adam had previously been healthy, sexually active, and free of any urinary difficulties whatsoever. Here he talks about his treatment decisions.

Q: When did you first discover that you might have prostate cancer?
Adam: It was seven years ago, when I was 45 years old. Previously, I had undergone a vasectomy. I had recently started a new job and was so wrapped up in it that I never went for my annual physical exam. My wife actually scheduled the appointment and forced me to go. And there was a jump in the PSA test that my general practitioner had been giving me since I was 40 years old. That threw up a red flag, and after that, one thing led to the next. *[Editor's note: Dr. Marc Garnick, the medical editor of this report, does not endorse PSA screening at age 40, nor do any major organizations that evaluate PSA testing. While the screening proved useful in Adam's case, there are no data to suggest that this practice is helpful for most men.]*

Q: Prostate cancer is typically considered a disease of older men. Was there a history of it in your family?
Adam: No, none at all, and I had no symptoms of cancer whatsoever.

Q: What was the increase in your PSA value?
Adam: When I was first tested at the age of 40, it was 0.5. Then three years later, it was 1.0, and when I was diagnosed two years after that, in 2007, it was 3.5.

Q: And so you were referred to a urologist?
Adam: That's right. He felt a hard bump on my prostate and it was targeted for a biopsy. It took about a week to get the results.

Q: Then what happened?
Adam: Well, I received a phone call from the doctor's office and I was told that the results did, in fact, show that I had a malignant tumor. After that, I was in complete shock. Again, I had no symptoms, I felt healthy, and I was very active. Not in a million years would I have thought there was anything like that wrong with me. I didn't hear much of what else he had to say after he told me that I had this cancer.

HARVARD MEDICAL SCHOOL   www.health.harvard.edu

Patient Perspectives *on* PROSTATE DISEASES

Key concepts: Hormonal therapy

Also known as androgen deprivation therapy, hormonal therapy treats prostate cancer by dramatically reducing levels of testosterone, which is a male hormone (or androgen) that fuels the growth of prostate cancer cells. It is a treatment option for men who

- have cancer that has spread beyond the prostate gland (metastatic disease)
- have cancer that is confined to the prostate but need to boost the effectiveness of radiation therapy or shrink the size of the prostate before brachytherapy (with radioactive seeds implanted in the prostate)
- have a rising PSA after initial treatment with surgery or radiation therapy, indicating that the cancer may have recurred.

Q: What were you told about your tumor?

Adam: The urologist sent me a lot of information, including that my tumor had a Gleason score of 9, meaning it was very aggressive and could possibly spread outside of the prostate gland.

Q: Did you search out other information on the Internet?

Adam: I did, and it flipped me out—everything I read suggested that I had slim chances of living a long life. Now when I talk to people with prostate cancer, I always say the same thing: the worst thing you can possibly do is go on the Internet. Prostate cancer is different for everyone, and until you get the specifics about your own disease, you can easily be led in the wrong direction.

Q: So how did your family react to this?

Adam: We all decided together that I needed to speak with other specialists. But the specialists we spoke to gave us a lot of conflicting opinions. There wasn't any real protocol for handling such an aggressive cancer in someone as young as me. But my father happened to know a medical oncologist who was able to clarify the options in a way that made sense to us. One message that came through loud and clear from our discussions with him was "Whatever you choose to do, do it fast."

Q: What diagnostic studies did you have?

Adam: I had a bone scan, an endorectal MRI scan [see "Key concepts: Endorectal MRI," page 28], and an abdominopelvic CT scan. Fortunately, they didn't show any signs that the cancer had spread.

Q: How did you and your family process all this information?

Adam: Two big questions stood out for all of us: We asked the medical oncologist, "How would you treat your own son if he was in this situation?" And we also wanted to know what could kill or stop the cancer from growing if it was spreading outside of my prostate. Based on those two questions, we decided the best thing to do would be to go with hormonal therapy and radiation [see "Key concepts: Hormonal therapy," at left].

Q: What about the option to go with surgery instead?

Adam: Well, we were initially thinking about surgery. But what kept us from doing that was the possibility that cancer cells might be spreading from the prostate even though we couldn't see them. Most men go with surgery because they think it's going to be easier, and because they want to get rid of the cancer as quickly as possible. By comparison, hormone and radiation treatments can take more than two years, and who wants to go through that? But I can't tell you how many men I speak to who got surgery and then wound up getting hormones and radiation anyway, because the cancer was still in their body. Lots of these men have problems with impotence and incontinence. Another factor was that my cancer was located near the nerves that control my ability to have an erection, and those nerves would have been removed with surgery. I was newly remarried, and my wife and I talked about this. We concluded that the priority was keeping me alive, and that we could worry about the sexual complications later, but this was definitely a secondary concern for me. So I went with hormonal therapy and radiation, and to this day, I believe I made the right choice.

Q: What was the treatment like?

Adam: The whole experience lasted for 26 months, and it was challenging. I got monthly shots of leuprolide [Lupron], and I was also given another hormonal treatment called bicalutamide [Casodex;

24   HARVARD MEDICAL SCHOOL   www.health.harvard.edu

Patient Perspectives on PROSTATE DISEASES

see "Key concepts: Medications used for hormonal therapy," at right]. Then after a few months, I got eight weeks of radiation treatment. For the first five weeks they irradiated my entire pelvic area, and then for the last three weeks they focused just on my prostate. The hormones put me through forced menopause as a male—my body became pear-shaped, and I lost the hair on my arms, legs, chest, and back. I was also extremely tired, and so I went to bed early every night. The whole idea of hormonal therapy is to shut down testosterone, so you also lose your sex drive and it's difficult to get an erection. I was given Viagra [sildenafil] and other treatments to help me, but the erections I did get were painful, and that was challenging for both my wife and me.

The radiation part was brutal. I had constant diarrhea after the first week, and I couldn't hold down foods that weren't bland. A few weeks into the process, I couldn't pee and needed medication for that. At one point, I collapsed with an intense migraine and was rushed to the emergency room. To this day, eating out remains very challenging for me.

Q: Did you speak with anyone else who had gone through a similar treatment?

Adam: I only wanted to speak with men who also had been diagnosed with a high Gleason prostate cancer during their 40s—nothing else mattered to me. So I networked and searched online all over the country, and I finally found three men who fit those criteria. One had literally just passed away, another was in pretty bad shape, and the third was in his late 60s and living in Vermont. He had undergone hormonal treatment for prostate cancer, and he was still living 20 years later. We had a nice conversation, and I felt better during my treatment knowing that he was still alive and doing well.

Q: Was your work or family life affected during this time?

Adam: I started a new career six months before I got diagnosed, and though it wasn't easy, I con-

---

Key concepts: Medications used for hormonal therapy

There are multiple classes of drugs that are used for hormonal therapy.

- Anti-androgens prevent testosterone from interacting with the testosterone receptor protein on prostate cancer cells. Drugs in this class include anflutamide (Eulexin), bicalutamide (Casodex), enzalutamide (Xtandi), nilutamide (Nilandron), and abiraterone (Zytiga, given with prednisone).
- LHRH agonists suppress testosterone indirectly, by inhibiting the production of a pituitary hormone—luteinizing hormone (LH)—that triggers testosterone production in the testicles. Drugs in this class include goserelin (Zoladex), histrelin (Vantas), leuprolide (Eligard, Lupron), and triptorelin (Trelstar).
- Gonadotropin-releasing hormone (GnRH) antagonists are another option for lowering testosterone by manipulating the pituitary—specifically, blocking the release of leuteinizing hormone. Degarelix (Firmagon) is the only drug in this class that is currently available in the United States.

---

tinued working every single day. I'd go to bed at 7 o'clock pretty much every night. My friends and family all knew that I might cancel plans last-minute because I was too tired. Everyone was cool with that. I was doing what I had to do to get through the treatment.

Q: How long did the side effects last?

Adam: I'd say it took two years for the hormones to clear out of my body. I've since gone back to having a very active sex life, which is terrific. And my body in general is back to normal. The only symptoms that linger from the radiation are diarrhea and some stomach pains that can be severe if I eat the wrong things. I kept food diaries during treatment and I recommend that others do too, so you know what makes you sick going forward.

Q: Any urinary difficulties?

Adam: Not really. Sometimes I have difficulty emptying my bladder all the way, but I can control that. I have no incontinence issues at all—never have, which is great. So, no, I'm feeling great right now, maybe just seven years older.

Q: What sort of follow-up are you having now?

HARVARD MEDICAL SCHOOL   www.health.harvard.edu

Patient Perspectives *on* PROSTATE DISEASES

2017 update:

Now 55 years old, Adam remains free of prostate cancer. His radiation-induced gastrointestinal problems (nausea and diarrhea) resolved roughly two years ago.

Adam: Well, for the first several years after finishing treatment I saw my doctor every three months for blood work and for a rectal exam. Since I was doing so well, he moved me to every four months, then every five months, and just recently, we switched to every six months. I'm looking forward to going once a year.

Q: Any advice or parting words for our readers?
Adam: The first thing I'd say is seek out multiple opinions, but be sure you see a medical oncologist. And do your homework. Come up with questions and try to listen to the different answers that doctors give you. Every prostate cancer differs according to so many variables, and you need to do what's right for you, not necessarily what's been right for other people. Today, I feel great—at 52 I'm still playing basketball, I'm swimming, and I'm getting ready for a 5K jog.

Jim and Terri Rogers

Jim and Terri Rogers are no strangers to medicine. Jim is a retired general and thoracic surgeon, and his wife, Terri, a retired operating room nurse. They have each spent more than 30 years working in hospitals and caring for patients. But that didn't make dealing with Jim's prostate cancer diagnosis much easier. Like most people confronted with the disease, they consulted multiple experts and went back and forth about the best treatment. Would robot-assisted laparoscopic prostatectomy or radiation therapy be most effective?

To help make the decision, the couple flew from their home on the West Coast to Boston so that Jim could undergo endorectal MRI, which wasn't offered in his area at that time. In some cases, advanced testing yields little concrete information, making it nothing more than technology for technology's sake. But for Jim, endorectal MRI helped pinpoint the location and likely extent of his tumor, ultimately showing him which path to choose.

In this 2008 interview, Jim and Terri share their experiences.

Q: What were the circumstances surrounding your prostate cancer diagnosis?
Jim: In November 2007, I had a general physical examination by my internist, and a PSA test revealed a PSA of 10 ng/ml. I had been having some urinary problems, so my doctor initially thought that the high PSA could be due to inflammation that accompanies prostatitis. So, I was placed on the antibiotic ciprofloxacin, or Cipro, 500 milligrams twice a day for three weeks. Then a follow-up PSA came back at 11 ng/ml, so on the advice of a friend who is a urologist, I was placed on Cipro twice a day for six more weeks. In April 2008, I had a third PSA test, which was 13 ng/ml. At that point, I consulted another urologist, who performed the biopsies and made the diagnosis.

Q: What did the pathology report show?
Jim: It was somewhat disquieting, revealing a Gleason 7—specifically, a 4+3 cancer—with perineural invasion, meaning the tumor was running along nerve cells, and could therefore be more prone to spreading. The other disturbing fact was that the tumor was present in five out of six biopsy samples, or cores, taken from the left lobe of the prostate.

Q: How did you react to the news?
Jim: I was absolutely stunned. I could not believe that I had prostate cancer. I'm well aware of the medical history of at least four generations of my family, and there hasn't been a single instance of prostate cancer. I attributed the 12 to 15 months of urinary symptoms that I had, which suggested a slight obstruction, to BPH.

Q: How old were you when the PSA test was done in November 2007?
Jim: I was 70.

Patient Perspectives on PROSTATE DISEASES

Q: *Had you ever had a PSA test before that?*
Jim: Many times, but the interval between the one in November and the one before that had been about two or three years.

Q: *Do you remember what your previous PSA was?*
Jim: I think it was in the range of 1.5 to 2 ng/ml, which wouldn't be considered abnormal for someone my age.

Q: *Terri, what was your reaction to the diagnosis?*
Terri: Well, when Jim came home after his physical in November and said his PSA was a little high, I wasn't particularly nervous. His internist didn't feel anything during the digital rectal exam, so he thought it was prostatitis. That was a little comforting. But when he had the second PSA done, I began to get nervous. We were in Costa Rica, and I said to Jim, "Maybe we should go back to the States and check into this." But a friend of ours, the second urologist Jim saw, didn't think things were really serious. He said to take the antibiotic for six weeks.

When we got home and Jim finished the second course of antibiotics only to have his PSA be even higher, I became very nervous. And when we finally got the diagnosis, I was devastated, at least at first. Then I was very angry with my husband. I had been harping on him for two years to see someone about his urinary problems. I'm a registered nurse, and I worked in an operating room for over 30 years. I knew that he had been having problems for almost two years. When I talked to him about it, he said, "It's just BPH."

Q: *What kind of urinary problems?*
Jim: My wife knew that my urinary stream had become weaker and that it took longer to "accomplish the mission."

Q: *What other tests did you have after the biopsy? What did the diagnostic work-up include?*
Jim: The diagnostic work-up following the biopsy included a bone scan, which temporarily sent up some red flags because there was dramatic activity in the eleventh rib on the left side. Subsequent CT scans and images of the ribs indicated that it was a fracture, not a problem associated with the cancer. I had a CT scan of the pelvis as well.

Q: *How did you get the information that you needed to decide what to do next?*
Jim: The first thing I did was consult the urologist who performed the biopsies. He recommended a prostatectomy. I asked him to set up an appointment with a radiation oncologist, and he did that. I met with that person, and we had a very thorough discussion. Initially, I had been leaning toward radiation therapy.

But then I learned about the robot-assisted procedure, the so-called Da Vinci procedure, which seemed like a more refined and elegant procedure than the standard prostatectomy. Even though the surgeon's fingers never enter the operating field, it's my personal belief that visibility is infinitely better. So at that point, I became quite anxious to move forward as a candidate for robot-assisted surgery. *[Editor's note: During robotic surgery, the surgeon sits at a console several feet away from the operating table and manipulates robotic arms fitted with tiny cameras and surgical instruments to locate and remove a diseased prostate gland.]*

Q: *But you came to Boston for another opinion. What made you, a well-respected surgeon in an area of the country known for top-notch medical care, travel across the country to see a doctor you didn't know?*
Jim: When a friend of mine, who is also a doctor, found out about the diagnosis, the first words out of his mouth were, "Oh, Jim, you have to see a friend of mine in Boston." I was receptive to the idea, recognizing that the more information I had up front, the better able I would be to make the correct treatment decision.

Q: *What additional studies did you undergo in Boston?*

HARVARD MEDICAL SCHOOL   www.health.harvard.edu

Patient Perspectives on PROSTATE DISEASES

Key concepts: Endorectal MRI

Magnetic resonance imaging (MRI) uses the electromagnetic properties of hydrogen molecules to collect information about organs and other tissues and converts that data into images. Because cancerous tissue has a different set of magnetic properties than normal tissue, it can stand out in pictures.

When performing MRI on the prostate, radiologists often use an endorectal coil. This is a thin wire that's covered with an inflated balloon and inserted into the rectum. The coil receives the magnetic waves, which are analyzed with a computer. The closer the coil is to the target tissue, the stronger the signal—and the better the pictures.

Jim: The trip to Boston was very informative. The doctor I saw voiced some skepticism about approaching my particular tumor with surgery. He also recommended endorectal MRI [see "Key concepts: Endorectal MRI," at left]. It seemed to me that the one piece missing in our decision making was that we didn't really have a clear handle on the extent of the tumor. The pelvic CT scan didn't show any evidence of lymph node involvement, but I thought the endorectal MRI would yield more information about the extent of the tumor. It wasn't being performed in my hometown at the time, so we made a second trip back to Boston.

Q: What did your endorectal MRI scan show?

Jim: It didn't show lymph node involvement. But it did show that the tumor was abutting the prostate capsule [the tissue that surrounds and covers the prostate gland]. It also looked like there could be a focus, or spot, of cancer in the left seminal vesicle. I take that particular finding with a grain of salt because it's always been my understanding that seminal vesicle involvement from prostate cancer is typically a direct extension of the tumor rather than a metastatic focus. But people with expertise in interpreting MRI results said there was a possibility that the seminal vesicle contained a separate tumor.

Q: And the MRI clinched your final decision?

Jim: Yes, and I was swayed toward external beam radiation. I realized that if there were positive margins [cancer cells in the edges of the tissue that was surgically removed, indicating that cancer likely remains in the patient following the surgery], I

would have to have radiation anyway. The incidence of urinary incontinence with both surgery and radiation is higher than with either treatment alone. Disease-free survival was my first goal. After that, the complication I wanted to avoid at nearly any cost was urinary incontinence.

Q: Why didn't you choose the robot-assisted prostatectomy?

Jim: I recognized that I had a fairly aggressive tumor, and after the MRI, we had clinical evidence that it at least abutted the prostate capsule. From my experience, I knew that there was probably microscopic disease outside the prostate capsule. My thinking was that I'd have a better chance of controlling the margins with external beam radiation than with surgery.

Q: You're a retired surgeon, and you know how the medical system works. You also have a close friend who is a doctor and was able to direct you to a specialist in Boston. What advice can you offer men who don't have these resources and don't know where to turn for help?

Jim: To make a decision about what treatment to pursue, I think it makes sense to get information from a medical center that focuses on the specific disease because that's obviously where the greatest expertise is going to be available. Now, if surgery is your chosen path, selecting a surgeon is a bit more difficult. Academic medical centers may be best when it comes to the overall approach to the problem, but the surgeon is an entirely separate matter. There are good surgeons and poor surgeons in academic medical centers, just as in community hospitals. But the layperson usually doesn't have access to that particular information.

Q: You are now home on the West Coast and under the care of a radiation oncologist. What's happening with your treatment?

Jim: I am taking two hormonal therapy medications—leuprolide [Lupron] and bicalutamide [Casodex; see "Key concepts: Medications used

28   HARVARD MEDICAL SCHOOL   www.health.harvard.edu

Patient Perspectives *on* PROSTATE DISEASES

for hormonal therapy," page 25]. That's resulted in a great many hot flashes each day, a common side effect. Aside from that, things are going well. My radiation therapy treatments aren't scheduled to start until early October.

Q: *Any parting comments or advice for our readers?*
Terri: It doesn't matter what your occupation or profession is or what your family history is. Prostate cancer can affect any man. Wives and partners really need to keep after the men in their lives

if they don't go to the doctor. Those regular visits are really important.

Q: *That's good advice. Do you have anything to add, Jim?*
Jim: Well, in the interest of keeping the remainder of the day harmonious, I'm going to say that perhaps husbands should listen to their wives. ♥

2017 update:

Now 80 years old, Jim remains disease-free and is pleased with his decision to have radiation as opposed to radical prostatectomy. He has regular PSA tests and physical exams of his prostate and spends much of his time together with his wife in Costa Rica.

Patient Perspectives on PROSTATE DISEASES

Prostate cancer treatment: Managing long-term complications

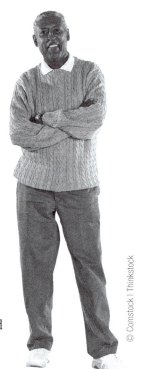

Prostate cancer treatments can be lifesaving, but they can also result in long-term side effects, such as urinary or fecal incontinence or sexual problems. Here we talk with three men about their own treatment complications. Tim Williams discusses his experience with erectile dysfunction and how a penile implant restored his sex life. Christopher Miller developed severe urinary incontinence that was finally resolved with a surgical procedure. Paul Doron developed a rare hardening of penile tissues, called Peyronie's disease, which results in painful, curved erections.

Tim Williams

In 1998, after his doctor discovered that his PSA level had been steadily rising, Tim Williams, then age 56, underwent a prostate biopsy. Days later, at 9:30 at night, his doctor phoned. Could Williams and his wife be in his office at noon the next day? Clearly, the news was not good.

Indeed, Tim had a fairly aggressive Gleason 3+4 cancer that needed treatment.

Ultimately, he chose surgery, and his PSA has been undetectable ever since. But like many men who have had a nerve-sparing prostatectomy, Tim was unable to have an erection firm enough for intercourse after the operation. In this 2010 interview, he talks about how he coped with erectile dysfunction (ED), the various options for men with post-surgery ED, and why he decided to get a penile implant.

Q: What was your erectile function like before you were treated for prostate cancer?
Tim: For the most part, it was fine. My wife and I shared an active sex life, and I didn't have any trouble getting or sustaining an erection.

Q: Did the possibility of ED or urinary incontinence factor into your decision to have surgery?
Tim: No, but I was well aware that surgery could cause them. My surgeon was very blunt about the risks. In fact, he said there was an 80% chance that I would be totally or partially impotent, and a 60% chance, at that time, that I would be incontinent. He did not hold back any information whatsoever.

Q: How involved was your spouse in your decision making?
Tim: My wife and I both felt that we should go with the treatment that offered the best chance of a cure, regardless of the side effects. At that point, surgery was the best option for someone of my age and health.

Q: What happened to your urinary and erectile function following surgery? What interventions did you pursue?
Tim: I did Kegels [see "Key concepts: Kegel exercises," page 31] for at least a month before I had surgery. After the catheter was removed, I was 99% continent.

Q: So you found Kegel exercises to be effective for preventing urinary problems?
Tim: I did. And yet I've had doctors at support groups say to me, "I'm not sure that doing them prior to surgery makes a difference." Regardless, I think men have to deal with the incontinence issue before they think about erectile function.

Q: So what happened with your erectile function?

HARVARD MEDICAL SCHOOL   www.health.harvard.edu

Patient Perspectives *on* PROSTATE DISEASES

Tim: When my erectile function was tested prior to my implant surgery in 2001, it was up to almost 70% of normal, but that's still not sufficient for penetration. Physicians and surgeons often ask men if they have any erectile function, but that's not the right question to ask. The question is whether there is enough erectile function for penetration.

Q: Viagra [sildenafil] was approved for the treatment of ED in 1998, the year you had your surgery. Did you try it?

Tim: My surgeon wanted me to wait at least five months before trying anything. After that, my wife and I went away for a long weekend, and my doctor gave me a prescription for Viagra. I started taking half a pill and then a whole pill, but it didn't do anything to improve my erectile function. The only thing I got from the pills was blue vision and a runny nose.

Q: What happened after you tried Viagra and found it ineffective?

Tim: My surgeon seemed reluctant to discuss it or talk about other treatment options, and we began to have a falling out. At one point, he actually said to me, "I don't understand why a man your age is so interested in sex." He was about 38 or 40 years old at the time. He made me feel like a "dirty old man" by suggesting that a man in his late 50s or early 60s had no business being interested in sex. That, of course, is ridiculous. I wonder if he has the same attitude now that he's in his 50s.

Q: Did you engage in any sexual activity over the next few years?

Tim: I did. I'm fortunate that my wife is still very much interested in sexual activity. It's an important part of our relationship. And besides, you just never know when you might get an erection. It can take a couple of years for erectile function to return following surgery.

Q: That's true. And there are many ways to be satis-

fied sexually without actually having intercourse.

Tim: Yes, we talk about this in my support groups. We're very blunt. You have fingers, you have lips, you have a tongue; there are any number of ways that you can satisfy your partner. Some men just don't know what else to do, so we talk about the options.

Q: How did the change in your sexual function affect your marriage?

Tim: My marriage remained pretty strong and positive. But from what I hear in my support groups, I'm well aware the loss of sexual function can cause significant problems in some relationships. Some men even blame their partners—make it someone else's fault.

Q: What happens to the men in your support group who suffer from ED? Do they have any characteristics in common?

Tim: I think a lot of the men become depressed. I urge them to talk about what's going on with their wives, their partners, their significant others. It's a problem that may take two to work out. Sometimes men in these circumstances feel as if they have no control over anything, including their sex lives. I'm sure that's what's behind some of the emotional problems surrounding ED.

Q: What made you decide to get a penile implant?

Tim: Compared with other approaches, it seemed like the simplest and most direct route to take. I had been reading about them and decided that I

Key concepts: Kegel exercises

The strength and proper action of your pelvic floor muscles are important in maintaining continence. Here's how to do basic pelvic muscle exercises, named for Arnold Kegel, the physician who first developed them:

1. Pretend you are trying to avoid passing gas. You will feel a contraction more in the back than the front, like you are pulling the anal area in.

2. Practice both short contractions and releases and longer ones (gradually increasing the strength of the contraction and holding it at your maximum for up to 10 seconds).

3. Repeat multiple times, several times a day.

For men, Kegels can help prevent post-void dribbling. But studies have not shown Kegel exercises alone to be particularly effective in preventing or treating incontinence that results from prostate surgery. That said, they cost nothing and are quite safe, so there is no harm in trying them.

HARVARD MEDICAL SCHOOL   www.health.harvard.edu

Patient Perspectives on PROSTATE DISEASES

was going to have the two-piece implant instead of a three-piece or malleable implant.

Q: How do the implants differ?

Tim: With the malleable implant, you have a permanent erection [see Figure 1, page 33]. It does not change shape; the length and girth remain the same. When you want to use it, you bend it up; when you don't want to use it, you bend it down. We joke that you could scare people in the locker room with it, but it is easy to use.

With an inflatable implant, either two-piece or three-piece, your partner might not even realize that you have one—they are that natural-looking and that natural-feeling. And you can be subtle enough when you're pumping it up that your partner may not be aware of what you're doing.

The two-piece implant never fully shrinks. That's because the fluid that creates the erection rests in chambers at the back of the implant and in a pump in the scrotum. When you squeeze the pump, the fluid is forced into cylinders in the penis. That's how you get an erection. When you are finished, you bend the penis and the fluid recedes back into the pump and into the chambers at the back of the implant. Since it has fewer parts, it's less likely to fail than a three-piece implant, and the surgery is also less complicated.

With the three-piece implant, you have the pump in the scrotum, cylinders in the penis, and a reservoir in the abdomen that holds the fluid. When you pump, you force the fluid from the abdominal reservoir into the cylinders. This implant looks more natural than the two-piece when it's deflated. And when it's inflated, you may get additional length and more girth. With the two-piece, the girth is pretty much fixed by the diameter of the cylinders that are installed during surgery.

Q: How long did the procedure take? What was your recovery like?

Tim: The surgery lasted just under two hours. I took Oxycontin [oxycodone] for three or four days,

and then the pain wasn't bad after that. I was driving by the sixth day, and on the eighth day I sat on a big feather cushion and used my lawn tractor.

There's no way to predict how long the pain will last. But everyone I've talked to has said, "It's worth it."

Q: How long did you have to wait until you could use the implant?

Tim: Generally, they want you to wait six weeks.

Q: Are you happy with your implant?

Tim: It took some getting used to, but I'm very pleased with it. My implant failed after four years, so I had another surgery to replace it. If and when this one fails, I would certainly get a third one.

Q: Did the implant make it easier or more difficult for you to urinate?

Tim: Actually, it made no change. But I've talked with 75 to 100 men who have had this surgery, and several of them have said that it tightens things up a bit, making any incontinence less of an issue. However, none of the doctors I've spoken with make that claim.

Q: Does an orgasm feel any different with an implant?

Tim: The sexual sensation is exactly the same as before the prostatectomy, but the orgasm is more intense. The consensus among the men who are open enough to talk about it is that orgasms last longer, too.

Another important point is that if your libido is low you can still perform. And there aren't any limitations on how often you can have sex.

Q: Did your self-image change after you got the implant?

Tim: Yes, without a doubt. I see a few men on a fairly regular basis who have been through the procedure, and we all agree that we walk taller, we look better, and we feel better. Our self-worth is higher, and that can't be discounted.

Figure 1. Penile implants compared

Semirigid (malleable) implant

Advantages
- Easy to use, especially for those with limited dexterity.
- Requires the least extensive surgery.
- Fewest parts, so less chance of malfunction.
- Least expensive type of implant.

Disadvantages
- Constantly firm.
- Somewhat harder to conceal than inflatable implants, but new designs make this less of a concern than in the past.

Comment
- For intercourse, lift the penis and make the rods as straight as possible.

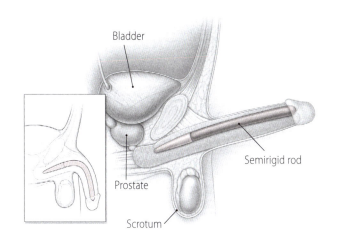

Two-piece inflatable implant

Advantages
- Penis looks more natural in erect and flaccid states than with the semirigid implant.
- Easier to operate than the three-piece implant.
- No abdominal incision.

Disadvantages
- Possibility of leakage or malfunction.
- The penis does not deflate as fully as with the three-piece implant.

Comments
- Squeeze and release the pump several times to move fluid into the penile cylinders.
- Bending and holding the penis causes the cylinders to soften.

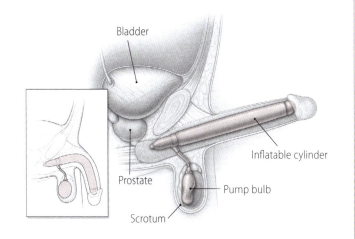

Three-piece inflatable implant

Advantage
- Acts and feels more like a natural erection than semirigid models.

Disadvantages
- Requires more manual dexterity than other implants.
- Possibility of leakage or malfunction.
- Most expensive type of implant.
- Requires the most extensive surgery of all implants.

Comments
- The inflate/deflate device is implanted in the scrotum. Squeeze the pump to inflate, and press the release valve to deflate.
- The fluid reservoir is implanted in the abdomen.
- Lockout valve can prevent unintended inflation.

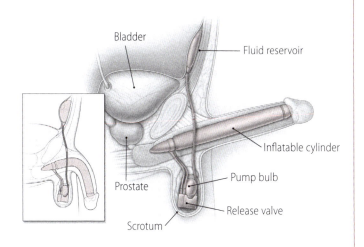

Patient Perspectives *on* PROSTATE DISEASES

2017 update:

Tim remains satisfied with his treatment decision and recommends penile implants to other men.

Q: How can the medical community's approach to ED be improved? What would have made your experience better?

Tim: Having spoken with hundreds of men, I've heard that many doctors will say, "See my colleague," or "See my nurse," or "See your general practitioner." They often give men the cold shoulder. They seem to want to cut out the cancer or irradiate it and be done with it. I think physicians need to become more comfortable in talking about this with their patients. And patients need to be more comfortable talking about impotence, too. As men, we need to under-stand that our sexuality is part of who we are and be comfortable with that.

Q: What advice do you have for a patient whose doctor seems less than helpful?

Tim: Walk away. Find someone else with an interest in ED.

Q: Any final points you'd like to make?

Tim: Getting a penile implant is something that men need to think about carefully because once the procedure is done, you can't have the implant removed and expect whatever function you still had to return. Also, find a physician who has done many of these implant procedures and has lots of experience.

Christopher Miller

Christopher Miller is a real estate agent who is married and has two sons. In 2002, at the age of 56, Christopher was diagnosed with prostate cancer. After a great deal of research and consultations with five doctors, Christopher decided to have a radical prostatectomy.

Although he considers the operation a success, in that it has apparently eradicated the cancer, Christopher struggled for almost two years to overcome persistent urinary incontinence. For much of that time, he felt ill-served by the medical community. In this 2007 interview, he discusses his experience.

Q: Can you share with our readers what was going through your mind when you learned you had prostate cancer?

Christopher: Like anyone else, I was surprised. You never think it's going to happen to you. I thought of things like: Is my family provided for? Are my financial affairs in order? Will my children be secure? Will I ever meet my grandchildren?

Of course, I was very concerned about my wife. We'd been married 32 years at that point, and I worried about what impact this would have on her. She's a very strong and good person, and she remained at my side every moment of the time. And that support proved to be invaluable.

Q: How many physicians did you see before making a treatment decision?

Christopher: As I recall, I saw two oncologists and three surgeons. They were all highly recommended. My wife and I were looking for a cure, and all of the information we were getting was that, given my set of circumstances, surgery was best. So then it was a question of who was going to perform the surgery.

Q: Did the doctors advise you about possible complications from surgery?

Christopher: They all explained that I might develop impotence or incontinence afterward. One reason that I finally chose the surgeon I did was because the complication rates he quoted were lower than the others'. He really believed that there was less than a 1% chance that I'd have an incontinence issue, and a 30% chance of impotence.

Q: And was that a deciding factor in your selection?

Christopher: Absolutely. I mean, here were all the big guns in town, and his numbers seemed like the best. I also asked around. And the feedback was, "He's got great hands." We knew that his bedside manner left a lot to be desired, but I thought, "Who needs bedside manner? Let's just get the best person, with the best hands, and let's get it done." And that's how we selected him.

Q: How did the operation go? And when did it become apparent that you might take longer to recover than you had been led to believe?

Christopher: The operation went fine. I went back to work very quickly, and in most respects I felt fine. I was incontinent immediately after surgery, but I was led to believe that the problem would straighten itself out within a few weeks or months. But it didn't.

Q: Did you share your concerns about incontinence with your surgeon?

Christopher: I did, during follow-up visits after the surgery. I probably visited him three to four times during the first six months after surgery. He told me the problem would get better, and for the first month or two, I believed that. But as time went on, nothing was getting any better.

And he didn't seem to care. In a typical visit, I waited a half-hour or an hour to see him for literally five minutes, and then he moved on to the next person. So I finally gave up on him.

Q: Could you tell our readers more about the problems you were experiencing?

Christopher: I had no problem at night, and I think for most people that's the case. But when I got up, I was going through anywhere from four to five pads a day. I used a high-absorbency pad that

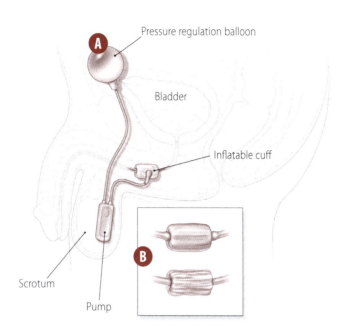

Figure 2. Artificial sphincter

An artificial sphincter is a surgically implanted device with three major components. An inflatable cuff surrounds the urethra; when inflated, it prevents urine from leaking out of the bladder. A pressure regulation balloon implanted in the lower abdomen (**A**) ensures that the cuff remains inflated until it is time to urinate. At that point, a man squeezes a pump located in the scrotum, which deflates the cuff enough so that urine can flow (**B**). The cuff then reinflates on its own.

tied around my hips on both sides, and I'd change it throughout the day. I tried doing Kegel exercises [see "Key concepts: Kegel exercises," page 31] to control the flow, but nothing worked. I was in trouble. I'm an active person. It was embarrassing, and it was the last thing I wanted to deal with.

Q: Was impotence an issue?

Christopher: Forget about sex! That was the last thing on my mind during this period. I knew I had to deal with the incontinence issue first.

Q: So what did you do?

Christopher: After about a year of waiting for this to get better, I consulted another surgeon. He recommended a sling procedure. I decided I would try this to see if it would make a difference. That was a mistake. It was a very difficult operation, more difficult than the radical prostatectomy.

Patient Perspectives on PROSTATE DISEASES

Q: *Did the second operation alleviate your incontinence?*

Christopher: No, everything was basically the same. That was a disappointment. After I told a friend about all my mishaps, he suggested I ask about having an artificial sphincter inserted. He'd heard it was very successful. I did consult one surgeon about it, but he hadn't done many of these operations.

So I was at a dinner, about a year and a half after I first developed incontinence, and I was talking to a woman whose husband was a prostate surgeon who had passed away. And I told her about my dilemma. She gave me the name and number of one of her husband's colleagues and told me to use her name when I called him. So I did.

When I met with him, he explained the artificial sphincter procedure to my wife and me. I was immediately comfortable with him. He performed the operation. And I must say it has changed my whole life for the better. I still wear a very tiny pad, just in case there's a leak when I bend a certain way or lift something, just for protection more than anything else. And I'm very happy with it.

Q: *Could you explain exactly how this works?*

Christopher: The surgeon inserts a small pump in the scrotum, which is attached to a sphincter cuff and a small balloon located near the belly button [see Figure 2, page 35]. When I feel the need to urinate, I go to the toilet, and I squeeze the pump in my scrotum with one hand. By pressing the pump, I deflate this cuff, and the pressure comes off the urethra. So at that point I'm able to urinate. Then probably 35 to 40 seconds later, the balloon fills back up. By then I've finished urinating, or if I haven't, I do it again.

Q: *Are you aware of this material in your scrotum when you're not using it?*

Christopher: Not unless I feel it with my hand. I can walk around, exercise, do everything I normally do, and I don't feel it. One challenge is riding a bike, because you need a flat seat so that your weight is better distributed, rather than concentrated in the middle. So I have to get another seat for my bike. But I can go out now and play football with my boys. I can do anything I want to do.

Q: *What was the recovery from this operation like, compared to the others you had?*

Christopher: It was probably a quarter as hard as the other two. It was nothing. I went in. I think I stayed overnight. And then I was back at work in a day or two.

Q: *What about potency? We haven't talked about that yet.*

Christopher: Once I dealt with the incontinence issue, when I felt that I was 98% back to normal, then I could really focus on the sexual part. I couldn't up to that point.

I'm not totally impotent. There are times when I can have intercourse without the aid of any chemical. But, I must say, it does help.

Q: *You've tried an erectile dysfunction drug?*

Christopher: Yes, but I'm not a "druggie" kind of person. If we want to go that route, which is very helpful in terms of creating more firmness, it means taking a pill and planning ahead. Sex is no longer spur-of-the-moment.

For me, the biggest change is that dealing with all of this enabled my wife and me to readdress our sexual life. And I think, as a man, you sort of think it's all about being hard and being up, and I think what has happened is that I'm now able to focus more on the other person, which I might not have been doing as well prior to this operation. It's made our sexual relationship deeper and stronger.

Q: *Knowing what you do now, what advice can you provide to people who are going to be reading this story?*

Christopher: I think you have to find a doctor who will give you the right information. The hurt for me was not necessarily that I developed incontinence. I just wished my original surgeon had been more honest with me. And I'd advise other men that they really need to question the numbers about side effects. If they know going into surgery that the likelihood of complications is high, then they're prepared.

What I can't understand, because surgeons have been performing prostatectomies for years, is why the information about incontinence and impotence isn't more accurate. There is information that is available, but it's not real. It's a shame. It's not right.

Q: Of course, in a typical office visit, sometimes the doctor can't address all these issues. There isn't time.

Christopher: But my surgeon didn't even ask. And where do I end up on his statistical map? I think urologists need to start dealing with this issue.

2017 update:

Now 72 years old, Christopher is still free of urinary symptoms, but questions his decision to have a radical prostatectomy.

Paul Doron

We interviewed a real estate professional—Paul Doron, age 53—about his experience with Peyronie's disease. This condition develops when patches of scar tissue called plaques form in the penis. These plaques aren't as malleable as normal tissues, and this leads to painful erections that curve downward, upward, or sideways. In some cases, the penis also becomes shorter. Men who have Peyronie's disease can find it difficult to have sex, and this can cause significant anxiety and stress.

Paul was diagnosed with Peyronie's disease five months after he had radical prostatectomy for prostate cancer, though it's not clear that his surgery was the cause. Some limited evidence, none of it confirmed, suggests that men who undergo this surgical procedure may have a higher risk of developing Peyronie's.

In this interview in early 2016, Paul discusses his experience with the condition.

Q: How and when did you learn you had prostate cancer?

Paul: It was two years ago, when I was 51. I'd been having my PSA checked during annual physical exams, and the level was slowly but steadily rising—between 2004 and 2010, it increased from 2.9 to 3.9. Then after a three-year gap, I had my PSA checked again, and this time the level had jumped to 6.2. So my doctor put me on a monthlong course of Cipro [ciprofloxacin], an antibiotic, to rule out infections in the urinary tract or prostate that can also elevate PSA. When we checked the level four months later,

in March 2014, it was 6.8. At that point, I had a biopsy and the results showed that I had Gleason 9 prostate cancer. I was stunned—it's very rare for a disease like that to show up in my age group.

Q. How did you go about choosing your treatment?

Paul: My local urologist recommended that I seek out a variety of opinions. Due to the aggressive nature of my cancer and my relatively young age, I did a great deal of research to understand the potential benefits and side effects of the various treatment options. I ended up seeing 17 doctors at four different hospitals. It appeared that my cancer was confined to the prostate gland, which meant that I was a good candidate for surgery. After consulting with my wife and family, I opted for open surgery to remove my prostate, and the results were about as good as I could have hoped for: the cancer hadn't spread to other tissues. Other than Peyronie's disease, I haven't had any other unexpected complications from my cancer treatment.

Q. Did you seek out advice on how to protect your sexual function during the immediate and long-term postoperative periods?

Paul: Yes. I was put on a course of Viagra prior to surgery and I've stayed on it ever since, at a daily dose of 25 milligrams. One doctor who specializes in sexual function recommended that I start using a vacuum pumping system for penile extension two weeks after my catheter was removed [see Figure 3, page 38]. He said that by bringing blood into my penis, the pump would help to keep tissues

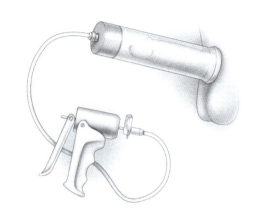

Figure 3. Vacuum pump

To achieve an erection, a man puts his lubricated penis into an airtight plastic cylinder attached to a handheld pump. Pumping air out of the cylinder creates a vacuum, which increases blood flow to the penis and causes an erection. An elastic band placed at the base of the penis maintains the erection.

healthy and substitute for the nighttime erections that I wouldn't be having. I was told that I should keep doing that until I had nighttime erections, and I used it every day for about half an hour. But I was never shown how to use the pump correctly. And when I used it for the first time, two weeks after my surgery, I had a painful mishap: for about 10 minutes, my penis was compressed in the pump's rubber sleeve and the compression worsened as I struggled to take the device off. I suspect that this incident may have contributed to my Peyronie's.

Q. When did you first start noticing a curve in your penis?
Paul: About four months after surgery, I noticed a curve to the left accompanied by noticeable shortening when I had an erection. I waited a month and it got worse, so I went to a sexual function specialist who told me I had Peyronie's disease.

Q. Had you ever heard of it before?
Paul: You know, I hadn't—I had no idea what it was. And when I started reading about it, I just felt sorry for myself. I couldn't believe that I now had to deal with this after everything else I'd been through.

Q. What was the initial treatment?
Paul: My new doctor told me to stop using the pump, and he recommended that I try penile traction therapy, which means you have to wear a device that gently pulls your penis in the opposite direction of the curve. But as with the pump, no one ever showed me how to use the traction device correctly. At the same time, I was given a drug called verapamil [Calan]. That's actually a blood pressure drug, but if it's injected into the penis, it can also help to break down scar tissue. I ended up having six treatments, each one involving at least 20 injections. It wasn't pleasant, but it's remarkable what you can get used to. And I wore the traction device for two to four hours a day, five to six days a week, for six months.

Q. Did you notice any improvement?
Paul: The initial curve to the left improved, but I also developed what looked like a new curve pointing in an upward direction. I've since found out that it was really an extension of the initial curve, so no, the treatment didn't appear to be helping much.

Q. So what happened then?
Paul: Unfortunately, the curve got worse. I've regained my potency with Viagra, and the curve in my penis isn't so bad that I'm unable to have sex. However, because the curve is more severe, my wife and I need to be careful when we do.

Q. What about pain? Was that a problem for you?
Paul: The pain during orgasm was very bad initially, and there was also some pain at the verapamil injection sites when I had an erection. The pain in both cases has gone away with time.

Q. What's happened with your Peyronie's disease more recently?
Paul: I recently saw a doctor who suggested that combining Xiaflex and traction would have a sig-

Patient Perspectives on PROSTATE DISEASES

nificantly positive effect [see "Key concepts: Treatment for Peyronie's disease," at right]. So, I'm back on traction, but now I'm doing it more aggressively: an average of six hours a day, seven days a week. I'm also keeping a daily log to help me stick with the treatment plan. I have been doing the traction for a month and I have seen some lengthening, but I am not yet sure if the traction is helping with the curvature. I expect to start Xiaflex in the next two weeks.

Q. What role has your wife played in your recovery?
Paul: My wife came with me to most of my doctors' visits so we could weigh my options together. Right after the surgery, she completely changed the way she cooks. I now eat a lot less dairy, sugar, flour, and animal protein, and a lot more organic fruits and vegetables. We only eat grass-fed meat.

Q. You've been through a great deal. Are there any parting thoughts you'd like to share with our audience?
Paul: I went to a sexual function doctor before my surgery with the goal of taking steps to protect the health of my penis until such time as I was able to have normal erections. But ironically, I now think the vacuum pump he told me to use either caused or contributed to my Peyronie's disease, maybe because I used it too quickly or used it incorrectly. I find it very disappointing that no one ever told me how to use the device, and that I was instead expected to follow the vague directions included in the packaging.

In hindsight, I think I would have been better off just sticking with Viagra and avoiding the vacuum pump so soon after surgery. The pump gave me instant erections, which was gratifying in the short term, but I was never advised about the poten-

Key concepts: Treatment for Peyronie's disease

The prognosis for men with Peyronie's disease varies. Most of the time, pain during erections lessens within a year or two. In some men, symptoms eventually go away without treatment, while in others, the condition stabilizes with the curvature remaining.

The FDA has approved only one medication, called collagenase clostridium histolyticum (Xiaflex), for treating Peyronie's disease. When injected directly into the penis, Xiaflex degrades the collagen in Peyronie's plaques, while sparing the different kind of collagen in blood vessels and nerve tissues. A clinician can then manipulate the affected area to stretch and elongate scarred tissues.

Xiaflex is approved specifically for men with a penile curvature of at least 30°. Treatments are given over four cycles, each comprising two Xiaflex injections into the affected area. Bruising, swelling, and pain are common side effects, but they generally resolve with time.

Doctors may also offer different treatments that have not specifically been approved for Peyronie's disease.

tial long-term consequences. It frustrates me that so many professionals were there to advise me on my cancer treatment, yet none told me about the possibility of Peyronie's disease after radical prostatectomy. So I did whatever I could do that was related to my cancer, but I didn't do what might have helped to prevent me from getting Peyronie's disease.

I would urge anyone with this diagnosis to be their own advocate and learn all they can about it. I would also recommend seeing a sexual function doctor. It's important to be gentle with your penis after radical prostatectomy, certainly for longer than two weeks. ◗

Late 2016 update:

At the time of his last doctor's visit, Paul was elated to hear that the cancer has not returned, as demonstrated by his undetectable PSA level. However, he remains distressed that he was not told that Peyronie's disease could result from radical prostatectomy and possibly from attempts at penile rehabilitation too soon after surgery.

Patient Perspectives *on* PROSTATE DISEASES

6 Finding social support

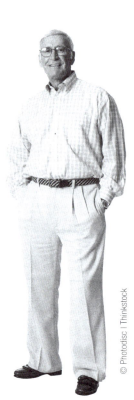

Men being treated for prostate diseases need caring support, whether from organized groups or friends and family members. Here we speak with Stanley Klein, who established one of the largest, longest-running prostate cancer support groups in existence today after he was diagnosed with aggressive, high-grade prostate cancer nearly 25 years ago. We also speak with two partners of men with prostate cancer about how they adapted and learned to take care of their respective partners (see "Two partners weigh in," page 43).

Stanley Klein*

The day after his radical prostatectomy in 1993, Stanley Klein, then 65 years old, heard a knock on the door to his hospital room. The visitor, an activist and prostate cancer survivor himself, invited Stanley to attend the first meeting of a new support group in Boston for men who were coping with the disease. Stanley knew that talking with others facing similar challenges would help him, but since he was still recovering from surgery, he demurred, at least temporarily.

Two months later, he attended a session of what would later become the Longwood Medical Area Prostate Cancer Support Group, one of the most successful organizations of its kind. Today Klein runs the organization, now called the Boston Prostate Cancer Support Group.

Experts often recommend that patients with prostate cancer attend a support group. Yet Stanley, who still runs the support group today, says that some men are hesitant to do so, even though it could help them make better informed treatment decisions and allay some fears and concerns. In this 2008 interview, he shares his story, explains the workings of his support group, and offers suggestions to men interested in launching their own successful support network.

*Although other interviews in this report use pseudonyms to preserve patients' privacy, Klein agreed to the use of his name.

Q: How did you find out that you had prostate cancer?
Stanley: A few days after I'd had my yearly check-up, my wife said to me, "Do you know your PSA?" I had no idea what PSA was. She had been reading a magazine and that very question was on the cover. When I had my check-up, I had a normal digital rectal exam, but I did not have a PSA test. Apparently, it was not regularly done in 1993. I went back to my primary care physician and asked for the test. Three days later, he called to say it must have been a faulty test because the score was so high. I had a PSA of 69 ng/ml, which was about 17 times higher than what was considered normal. So we repeated the test, and it was 69 again.

I had a biopsy, and it confirmed a very aggressive cancer—the Gleason was 5+4, for a total score of 9. My urologist and primary care physician both recommended surgery, so I had a radical prostatectomy. When the pathology report came back, it said there were positive margins, meaning some cancer was left behind. So four months after the radical prostatectomy, I had seven weeks of external beam radiation.

Q: And you've been fine ever since?
Stanley: That is correct. It's been almost 15 years, and my PSA is still basically undetectable—less than 0.1 ng/ml.

HARVARD MEDICAL SCHOOL   www.health.harvard.edu

Patient Perspectives on PROSTATE DISEASES

Q: *What side effects did you experience as a result of your treatment?*

Stanley: The urinary incontinence started right after the surgery. And of course, all sexual function was gone; having both a radical prostatectomy and radiation eliminated any hope of getting normal erections. My wife was so worried about me during the surgery that she begged me not to have any more operations. So I use a vacuum pump instead of a penile implant. Actually, I did not want to have any more surgery, either!

Q: *How did you end up heading the Longwood Medical Area Prostate Cancer Support Group?*

Stanley: My urologist started the group at the Deaconess Hospital, which is now part of the Beth Israel Deaconess Medical Center. A few months after my surgery, he and another prostate cancer survivor asked me if I would share the role of patient coordinator. I agreed. At that time, six to eight men attended.

After a few months, I realized that there were no other support groups for prostate cancer survivors nearby, but there were many other hospitals. So I made an appointment with the chief of urology at Beth Israel Hospital, told him about the new group, and asked if he would join us. He immediately agreed, and the meetings alternated between Beth Israel and the Deaconess, which later merged. Then I went to Brigham and Women's Hospital and Dana-Farber Cancer Institute. They both agreed to participate, too. We changed the name to the Longwood Medical Area Prostate Cancer Support Group *[Editor's note: It's now called the Boston Prostate Cancer Support Group]*, and we soon had 30 to 35 people showing up at each meeting. Then I helped facilitate a second support group at another hospital, and I was a guest speaker and consultant for a support group at a third hospital. But within a few years, they disbanded, and they joined us.

We have three subgroups: one to discuss erectile dysfunction and urinary incontinence, another to discuss prostate cancer diagnosis and treatment, and a third for men with advanced and metastatic cancer.

From 7 to 8:30 p.m., everyone gathers in the main meeting room. Nine times a year, we have a speaker. The other three times a year, people ask any questions they want, and others try to answer. Usually, we have our physician coordinator, a medical oncologist, on hand to answer questions, too.

Q: *What has your role been?*

Stanley: My role is to obtain speakers, reserve conference rooms, order refreshments, obtain parking validation stickers, answer phone calls, and get our monthly flyers printed, mailed, and posted at the local hospitals.

I learned that I had to have a competent "staff." We had to cover the three subgroups, so I found four people, with the fourth to cover in case one of the others couldn't attend. I can cover a subgroup, too, if necessary.

Q: *You've been personally involved as a peer counselor, too, correct?*

Stanley: Well, I try to guide the men with the knowledge that I have gathered from my own research and listening to many other people. We discuss topics that other groups seem to stay away from, such as side effects and recurrence. Men sometimes call when they've just been diagnosed and they don't know who to see. I try to give advice—not medical advice, of course, but information on the type of doctor to see for their particular situation.

Q: *What concerns do men and their spouses or partners share during the group sessions or when you talk with them individually?*

Stanley: Their concerns depend on how long they've been dealing with the cancer. If a man has just been diagnosed, he's confused as to which treatment to have, and usually he's poorly informed. He's looking for basic information.

If a man has advanced or metastatic prostate cancer, his main concern is to live, hopefully with a

HARVARD MEDICAL SCHOOL www.health.harvard.edu

Patient Perspectives on PROSTATE DISEASES

decent quality of life. Nothing else is important. He wants to live long enough to see his son graduate from college, or attend his daughter's wedding.

If a man is out of immediate danger of dying, his greatest concern is quality of life. He wants to learn how to overcome incontinence and impotence and learn what he can do to avoid a recurrence. Should he change his diet? Should he take supplements? Should he exercise?

Q: What role can families play?
Stanley: They can help psychologically. Many women and adult children attend the support groups, sometimes without their mate or father because he is too embarrassed to let anyone know he's got prostate cancer. So they come to learn and then bring information home.

Q: How do you help so many people who are dealing with different issues? How do you make meetings relevant to everyone?
Stanley: I bring lots of articles from journals and other sources. We spread them out on tables so that the men can read about any topic they want. The subgroup leaders and I try to answer other questions. And then the speaker talks about his topic. Somehow, we manage to have something that helps everyone.

Q: What are the advantages of attending a support group?
Stanley: A good support group is invaluable. Often the people who attend have done some research on their own. That gives them the basics, but support groups can provide more information and answer questions people never thought to ask!

Support groups also offer psychological support to both the man and his family. When I point out men who are 10-year cancer survivors, or 12-year cancer survivors, or 14-year survivors, newly diagnosed patients have hope. You'd be amazed to see how their countenance changes. When someone who's been recently diagnosed

sees that, he realizes, "Gee, maybe I won't die next week."

We alert the men to possible side effects or problems that they may not be aware of and possible solutions. Also, we correct misinformation. Sometimes I can't believe what a newly diagnosed person says! I'm not blaming him; he's just heard something from a friend, who heard it from a friend, who heard it from a friend.

The subgroups offer specialized information. If a man wants to learn about overcoming erectile dysfunction after cancer treatment, he can come to our subgroup on impotence and incontinence. We show men the devices that are available to help them have an erection—the vacuum system, penile implants, and injections. And we have people speak on those topics.

I have two sayings that sum up what a support group is. The first one is "Sharing is caring." The second one is "Learn to cope through knowledge and hope." A good support group does both.

Q: How does your group differ from others? What makes it so popular?
Stanley: I'm blessed to be in an area where there are so many hospitals and specialists. That makes it relatively easy to get speakers on a wide range of topics.

I also have a reputation for questioning speakers if I think they've left out key facts. I will refer to a specific article in a particular journal, for example. I do it very politely, of course, but people realize that they're getting a balanced, accurate picture at our meetings. When they leave, I don't want them to have any misconceptions.

We have male and female licensed clinical social workers at our meetings, and we're the only group in New England that offers sessions for women.

Q: What are women most concerned about?
Stanley: Their main concern is obviously their mate. They want him to live, and they want him to be happy and productive. About 30% of men have some degree of incontinence, and they are embar-

continued on page 44

Patient Perspectives on PROSTATE DISEASES

Two partners weigh in

As with any serious disease, when prostate cancer strikes, its reach goes beyond the patient. Entire families feel the impact. But because treatment for prostate cancer can affect continence and sexual functioning, it can hit at the core of romantic, intimate relationships.

Re-establishing intimacy after treatment requires honest communication about each person's needs. Even when couples do become intimate again, they can struggle because the experience is often quite different from what they were used to. Sex may no longer be spontaneous, especially if a man needs to use injections or a vacuum pump to get an erection. One or both partners might be turned off if a man leaks or dribbles urine in bed or during foreplay. And all of this can lead to frustration, confusion, and anger.

Numerous patients and their partners say that the key to success is, not surprisingly, communication—and lots of it. People who aren't comfortable talking with their partner about erections and orgasms can try working with a clinician or therapist who can help get the conversation started. There are also publications from the American Cancer Society, available online at www.cancer.org, and other organizations.

To help prepare patients and their partners for the changes prostate cancer can impose on a relationship, we spoke in 2009 with two women whose partners had a radical prostatectomy.

Catherine Golden's story

We asked Catherine how she and her husband of 16 years, Tom, decided on a radical prostatectomy to treat his prostate cancer. She replied bluntly, "Our priorities were breathing, continence, and sex, in that order. We were both in agreement on that." As they investigated the various treatments, they kept looking back at their priorities.

"We read everything we could get our hands on," Catherine recalled. "We knew more about prostate cancer and the treatments than Tom's primary care doctor! But we had a bias toward surgery. We just wanted the cancer out. We've had lots of family members who've had cancer, and this had been their approach. We never talked to a radiation oncologist about radiation therapy because we knew what the possible side effects were. At that time, in 2004, radiation wasn't as focused as it is now, and we really wanted to avoid rectal problems and fecal incontinence, which were more likely with radiation."

Tom ended up needing radiation therapy anyway. After surgery, the pathology report came back showing positive margins, and his Gleason score was revised from a 3+3 to a 3+4, indicating that the cancer was a bit more aggressive than originally thought. The lymph nodes were clear, but his PSA never dropped to zero, as it should have if the cancer had all been removed. Tom's doctor recommended radiation, which Tom started several months later, after his urinary continence returned. It worked, and his PSA has been nonexistent ever since.

Tom's potency, however, still has not returned. "There's nothing wrong with his libido," Catherine says, "so it really bothers him that he can't have intercourse. I miss it, too, because he was very good. But we cuddle as often as we always have, and he helps me achieve orgasm. It's different, but if it were a choice between this and not having him at all, well, there's no contest."

Even so, Tom has sought solutions for his erectile dysfunction. He tried penile injections at a specialist's office, but the result paled in comparison to "the real thing," and the needles proved to be a mental hurdle. "We talked about a penile implant [see Figure 1, page 33], and he said he would do it for me, but I told him not to go there," Catherine says. "If he wants an implant and decides that is what he needs to be happy, that's fine. But I don't want him to get an implant for me."

One thing Tom and Catherine regret is that no one talked with them about using sildenafil (Viagra) or another PDE-5 inhibitor right after Tom's surgery. "We didn't expect to have sex right away," explains Catherine, "but because these drugs are vasodilators, they open up the blood vessels, increase blood and oxygen flow, and promote healing. Maybe that would've changed things, but that wasn't the thinking five years ago."

Catherine's relationship advice for other couples: talk. "Couples have to be open to talking about sex. What does each person want? What are their needs? Things are going to be different, but if you can't talk about it, you can't fix it. And keep saying 'I love you.'

"My other recommendation," Catherine continues, "is not to second-guess your decisions. There's so much information out there. It can be hard to cull through it and figure out what you really need to know, so consider going to a support group meeting before making a choice. Listen to people who have gone through it. People at the group meetings tend to be more candid than physicians—and you'll feel like you have more control over the process."

2017 update: Tom has accepted that he is impotent and does not want treatment for it.

continued on page 44

HARVARD MEDICAL SCHOOL   www.health.harvard.edu

Patient Perspectives *on* PROSTATE DISEASES

continued from page 43

Kate Hill's story

Kate, 48, met her boyfriend, David, at a friend's Thanksgiving dinner in 2008. The two had an almost instant connection and started dating. Because they spent so much time talking about their lives and discovering all that they had in common, they quickly grew close. So Kate didn't find it odd when David, 54, told her on their first date that he had been treated for prostate cancer four years earlier.

"I told him that my mother was about to have a mastectomy, and he said that he had been through prostate cancer," she recalled. "Maybe it was a little early in the relationship, but he was so matter-of-fact about it and needed so little prompting that it wasn't an uncomfortable discussion at all. So, I knew before our first sexual encounter and didn't think twice about it."

David revealed that he had opted to have his prostate removed. The cancer, which was detected through screening, was small, and its location meant that the nerve bundles could be left intact. After the operation, he suffered from incontinence for a few months, and he had to wear a pad when he went running. He also started taking tadalafil (Cialis), but after a few months, that wasn't necessary. He could have an erection without it.

"He also told me that he has a dry orgasm. It never occurred to me that a man would not ejaculate after prostate surgery, but I thought it was wonderful," said Kate with a laugh. "He was the perfect man. No cleanup would be necessary, and I wouldn't have to reach for the box of tissues afterward!"

Her sense of humor probably helped ease any tension after they tried to have intercourse for the first time. "Even though he said that he'd never had a problem before, he wasn't able to sustain an erection with me. I didn't know what to think because he seemed so aroused. But he also seemed frustrated and unnerved. He kept saying he wanted to share that experience with me, and he seemed genuinely surprised by his inability to stay hard."

More attempts at intercourse, all unsuccessful, followed. "I thought he was putting too much pressure on himself and that it was just performance anxiety," said Kate. "I also started thinking that maybe he still had feelings for a previous partner, but he said that wasn't it. And he said I must have thought he was lying to me about his ability to have an erection.

"In retrospect, there was probably too much focus on the lack of an erection and orgasm," said Kate. "I reassured him that I was enjoying the intimacy we had together. He was enjoying my orgasms if not his own!"

David decided to try taking tadalafil again, because he responded well to it in the months after his surgery. It worked. "After that first success, it was sheer relief for him," said Kate. "I think he felt the need to prove himself and to show that he was still young, sexy, and capable. The sexual piece is part of his identity.

"After we 'accomplished the mission,' he thanked me for my patience. That made me realize that he thought I might give up on the relationship, but I honestly never considered that. I certainly would've felt that I was missing out on something if there wasn't any physical intimacy; I think that's an integral part of a relationship. But his having an erection wasn't a 'make or break' for me."

Kate wonders whether David will continue with the tadalafil regularly if he needs to—she wants him to but is afraid to ask. She doesn't want him to think she wouldn't stay with him if he stops taking it. "It's difficult because the relationship is so new, and we're both finding our way. It is a sensitive subject, but this will be a good test of how we communicate about all kinds of things," she says.

2017 update: Unavailable.

---

continued from page 42

rassed about that. Some of them want to go into a shell. They don't want to go out to a movie, or a party, or a wedding. The women talk about how to encourage their husband or partner to socialize, how to tell him that the world hasn't come to an end, that he's still a man, that he's still loved, and that he can get help. They talk about how to have a sexually satisfying relationship without having intercourse. And they talk about how to prevent their men from becoming too despondent. Believe it or not, that's one of the biggest problems! Unlike most men, women tend to be interested in the psychological aspects of the disease. Men are interested in the how-to: How can I be treated? How can I overcome my side effects? How can I prevent a recurrence? How can I have an erection?

Q: *How do you keep people engaged and coming back month after month?*

Stanley: Hundreds and hundreds of people have told me they've learned more from the support group than from all the books they've read and all their conversations with their doctors. They keep coming back until their condition has stabilized. At that point, they often drop out. I hope I never see them again. But a few years later, some come back, not because I'm a nice, friendly guy, but because they've had a recurrence and they feel they will benefit.

Other people attend when we are going to cover certain topics—urinary incontinence, for example—or have a speaker with expertise in a particular area, such as a medical oncologist or someone who specializes in sexuality. Some people just keep coming because they always want to learn and support new members.

Q: Do you have any advice for others who may be thinking about establishing a support group in their area?
Stanley: Obtain speakers who are as objective as can be. This is very important. Also, I try to avoid inviting primary care physicians to speak, not because they aren't nice people, but because they usually don't have the specialized knowledge the men are looking for. Speakers should also focus on what will help people now. Sometimes, they'll want to talk about their work in mice and how it might lead to a new drug one day. Their work might help all of the mice in the world, but the people in the audience want help today.

Q: Any final comments?
Stanley: I know people have great concerns. I just try to give them hope, encouragement, and the technical information they need to make the decisions that are right for them. ⬮

2017 update:

Now 90 years old, Stanley credits the treatment he had decades ago with saving his life. He hasn't needed additional cancer therapy, but his urinary incontinence problems have never resolved. Moreover, Stanley underwent radiation therapy several months after surgery. About 12 years later, he developed fecal incontinence—a side effect from the treatment that he still lives with today. He says radiation delivery has since become more precise, so that treated men aren't at such high risk for fecal incontinence as they once were. Stanley recommends that men know who will perform their radical prostatectomy before the operation takes place. He also says that men should be sure to check with a medical oncologist who can provide an independent assessment of the available treatment options.

Resources

Organizations

American Urological Association (AUA)
1000 Corporate Blvd.
Linthicum, MD 21090
800-828-7866 (toll-free)
www.auanet.org

The AUA is a professional association for the advancement of urologic patient care. It helps physicians and patients stay current on the latest research and practices in urology. The AUA also provides a range of services, including publications, research, meetings, and guidance on health policy.

Harvard Health Publishing (HHP)
Harvard Medical School
4 Blackfan Circle, 4th Floor
Boston, MA 02115
877-649-9457 (toll-free)
www.health.harvard.edu
www.harvardprostateknowledge.org

A division of Harvard Medical School, HHP publishes subscription newsletters, in-depth health reports on a variety of topics, and books. In 2009, HHP launched the free Harvard Prostate Knowledge website, which includes articles on prostate diseases from the company's publications as well as patient perspectives and brief summaries of groundbreaking prostate research.

National Cancer Institute (NCI)
Office of Communications and Education
9609 Medical Center Drive, Room 2E-532
Bethesda, MD 20892
800-422-6237 (toll-free)
www.cancer.gov
Office of Cancer Survivorship:
www.cancercontrol.cancer.gov/ocs

This government agency, part of the National Institutes of Health (NIH), conducts and sponsors research on all types of cancer. Operators can answer questions, provide informational booklets and brochures on prostate cancer, and make referrals to local resources. The NCI also offers the latest information about cancer clinical trials, including their locations. The website provides online information for patients, health professionals, and the public.

Prostate Cancer Foundation
1250 Fourth St.
Santa Monica, CA 90401
800-757-2873 (toll-free)
www.pcf.org

This philanthropic organization funds prostate cancer research. Its website offers general information about prostate cancer; a list of resources for patients needing financial assistance; help finding a doctor or treatment center; and support for patients and families.

Prostatitis Foundation
1063 30th St., Box 8
Smithshire, IL 61478
www.prostatitis.org

This nonprofit organization provides information about prostatitis and sponsors research into this condition.

Us TOO International Prostate Cancer Education and Support Network
2720 S. River Road, Suite 112
Des Plaines, IL 60018
630-795-1002
Support hotline: 800-808-7866 (toll-free)
www.ustoo.org

This large network of independent support groups provides information, counseling, and education for prostate cancer patients and their families. To find the chapter nearest you, or for more information on prostate cancer treatment options, call the hotline or visit the website.

Newsletter

Harvard Men's Health Watch
This monthly newsletter is written specifically for men, to help them lead healthier, longer lives. Topics include prostate disease, heart disease, nutrition, exercise, erectile dysfunction, and much more. To order, go to www.health.harvard.edu/mens.

Harvard Special Health Reports

The following publications from Harvard Medical School provide more information about some of the topics in this report. To order, call 877-649-9457 (toll-free) or go to www.health.harvard.edu.

2018 Annual Report on Prostate Diseases: Covering advances in the diagnosis and treatment of prostate cancer, benign prostatic hyperplasia, erectile dysfunction, prostatitis, and related conditions
Marc B. Garnick, M.D., Editor in Chief
(Harvard Medical School, 2018)

This report, from the medical editor of *Patient Perspectives on Prostate Diseases*, gives in-depth coverage of prostate problems, including cancer. It describes the latest studies and treatments. Includes information on risk factors for cancer, biomarkers that can help patients avoid unneeded biopsies, comparisons of treatments, and more.

Better Bladder and Bowel Control: Practical strategies for managing incontinence
May M. Wakamatsu. M.D., Joseph A. Grocela, M.D., and Liliana Bordeianou, M.D., Medical Editors
(Harvard Medical School, 2017)

This report covers medical and surgical treatments for urinary and fecal incontinence, including less invasive procedures that can be done on an outpatient basis. It also includes a special section on coping with urinary incontinence through a variety of devices and products, such as absorbent underwear and collection devices.

Patient Perspectives on PROSTATE DISEASES

Resources *continued*

Erectile Dysfunction: How medication, lifestyle changes, and other therapies can help you conquer this vexing problem
Michael P. O'Leary, M.D., M.P.H., Medical Editor
(Harvard Medical School, 2016)

This report offers a comprehensive review of the many causes of erectile dysfunction and the most effective male importance treatment options. It also includes information on sex therapy and involving your partner in treatment.

Life After Cancer
Ann Partridge, M.D., Medical Editor
(Harvard Medical School, 2017)

Cancer survivorship means that you have survived the first, active phase of treatment and been able to resume your life. Your chal-lenges have shifted—but they have not disappeared. This report helps you deal with long-term and late effects of cancer treat-ment, cope with cancer's aftermath, and create a survivorship care plan.

Sexuality in Midlife and Beyond
Jan Leslie Shifren, M.D., and Suki Hanfling, M.S.W., L.I.C.S.W., Medical Editors
(Harvard Medical School, 2015)

Advancing years affect the body, mind, and emotions—and, inevitably, your sex life. But you can overcome these challenges and develop a better, more satisfying sex life. This report details the treatments, medications, and self-help techniques that can resolve common sexual problems. A special section deals with sex therapy.

HARVARD MEDICAL SCHOOL   www.health.harvard.edu

Glossary

active surveillance: A strategy for managing prostate cancer in which the patient is regularly examined but is not treated until the disease shows signs of worsening.

acute urinary retention: An inability to squeeze any urine past the enlarged prostate because the bladder has become distended and its muscular wall has weakened.

alpha blocker: A medication used to treat high blood pressure and benign prostatic hyperplasia and often prescribed for chronic prostatitis.

androgens: The male hormones, particularly testosterone and dihydrotestosterone.

anti-androgen: A type of drug that blocks the growth-promoting influence of androgens on the prostate gland and prostate cancer cells.

benign prostatic hyperplasia (BPH): A noncancerous enlargement of the prostate that can interfere with urination.

biopsy: A procedure in which small samples of tissue are removed for analysis under a microscope.

brachytherapy: A form of radiation treatment using seeds or pellets of radioactive material, which are implanted in the prostate to destroy cancer cells.

catheter: A narrow, flexible tube inserted into the urethra and up into the bladder to allow passage of urine when someone is unable to urinate.

core: A piece of tissue obtained in a biopsy of the prostate.

cryotherapy: A surgical procedure that eliminates abnormal tissue by freezing it.

digital rectal examination (DRE): A screening test in which the physician inserts a gloved finger into the rectum to examine the prostate for abnormalities.

endorectal MRI: Magnetic resonance imaging done with a coil (consisting of a probe and an inflatable balloon) inserted into the rectum. The test helps doctors assess cancer spread and local invasion.

erectile dysfunction (ED): A more specific term for impotence that refers to the inability to have and maintain an erection sufficient for intercourse.

fecal incontinence: The inability to control bowel movements, resulting in involuntary discharge of liquid or solid feces.

5-alpha reductase: An enzyme that converts testosterone to dihydrotestosterone. The latter stimulates prostate growth.

Gleason score: A numerical grade that describes prostate cancer based on its aggressiveness.

GnRH antagonists: Gonadotropin-releasing hormone antagonists. Like LHRH agonists, these drugs treat prostate cancer by blocking the release of luteinizing hormone, but without a temporary surge in testosterone.

hormonal therapy: Treatment for prostate cancer (with either drugs or surgery) that is intended to reduce or eliminate the supply of male hormones to the prostate and distant cancer sites, thereby slowing cancer growth.

impotence: Erectile dysfunction.

laparoscopic surgery: A surgical approach in which a procedure is carried out with tiny instruments inserted through small openings in the skin.

LHRH agonists: Drugs used to treat prostate cancer by preventing the secretion of luteinizing hormone–releasing hormone (LHRH), which prompts testosterone production.

luteinizing hormone: A hormone released from the brain that controls the production of androgens by the testes.

lymph nodes: Small, specialized clusters of tissue that help fight infections and capture cancer cells that have moved out of a given tissue or organ.

magnetic resonance imaging (MRI): A test that relies on magnetic fields to visualize abnormalities in the body.

margin: An edge of normal-looking tissue surrounding an excised tumor. The presence of cancer in the margins can be confirmed under a microscope after the tumor is removed.

medical oncologist: A physician who specializes in chemotherapy, hormonal therapy, biological therapy, and targeted therapy for cancer; usually the main health care provider for someone with cancer.

metastasis: The spread of cancer throughout the body, beyond the organ or tissue in which it originated.

nanograms per milliliter (ng/ml): A measurement for a small quantity of a substance in liquid; 1 ng/ml means one-billionth of a gram (454 grams make 1 pound) in one-thousandth of a liter (1 liter is approximately 1 quart).

nerve-sparing: In prostatectomy, the surgical approach that seeks to preserve the nerves necessary for potency.

oncologist: A physician who deals with the diagnosis and treatment of cancer. There are three types of oncologists—medical oncologists, radiation oncologists, and surgical oncologists.

open prostatectomy: A surgical procedure in which prostate tissue is removed through an incision in the abdomen.

PDE5 inhibitors: Drugs that block PDE5, an enzyme that breaks down erection-producing chemicals. These drugs can help a man achieve and maintain an erection.